Clinical Pocket Manual

Critical Care

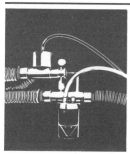

NURSING85 BOOKS™
SPRINGHOUSE CORPORATION
SPRINGHOUSE, PENNSYLVANIA

Clinical Pocket Manual™ Series

PROGRAM DIRECTOR
Jean Robinson

CLINICAL DIRECTOR
Barbara McVan, RN

ART DIRECTOR
John Hubbard

EDITORIAL MANAGER
Susan R. Williams

EDITORS
**Lisa Z. Cohen
Kathy E. Goldberg
Virginia P. Peck**

CLINICAL EDITORS
**Donna Hilton, RN, CCRN, CEN
Joan E. Mason, RN, EdM
Diane Schweisguth, RN, BSN**

COPY SUPERVISOR
David R. Moreau

DESIGNER
Maria Errico

PRODUCTION COORDINATOR
Susan Powell-Mishler

Material in this book was adapted from the following series: Nurse's Reference Library, Nursing Photobook, New Nursing Skillbook, Nursing Now, and Nurse's Clinical Library.

Library of Congress Cataloging-in-Publication Data

Main entry under title:

Critical care.

(Clinical pocket manual)
"Nursing86 books."
Includes index.
1. Intensive care nursing—Handbooks, manuals, etc. I. Springhouse Corporation. II. Series.
[DNLM: 1. Critical Care—handbooks. 2. Critical Care—nurses' instruction. WY 39 C934]
RT120.I5C73 1986 616'.028 85-27667
ISBN 0-87434-010-1 (pbk.)

CONTENTS

Nursing86 Books™

CLINICAL POCKET MANUAL™ SERIES
Diagnostic Tests
Emergency Care
Fluids and Electrolytes
Signs and Symptoms
Cardiovascular Care
Respiratory Care
Critical Care
Neurologic Care
Surgical Care

NURSING NOW™ SERIES
Shock
Hypertension
Drug Interactions
Cardiac Crises
Respiratory Emergencies
Pain

NURSE'S CLINICAL LIBRARY™
Cardiovascular Disorders
Respiratory Disorders
Endocrine Disorders
Neurologic Disorders
Renal and Urologic Disorders
Gastrointestinal Disorders
Neoplastic Disorders
Immune Disorders

NURSING PHOTOBOOK™ SERIES
Providing Respiratory Care
Managing I.V. Therapy
Dealing with Emergencies
Giving Medications
Assessing Your Patients
Using Monitors
Providing Early Mobility
Giving Cardiac Care
Performing GI Procedures
Implementing Urologic Procedures
Controlling Infection
Ensuring Intensive Care
Coping with Neurologic Disorders
Caring for Surgical Patients
Working with Orthopedic Patients
Nursing Pediatric Patients
Helping Geriatric Patients
Attending Ob/Gyn Patients
Aiding Ambulatory Patients
Carrying Out Special Procedures

NURSE'S REFERENCE LIBRARY®
Diseases   Definitions
Diagnostics   Practices
Drugs   Emergencies
Assessment   Signs and Symptoms
Procedures

NURSE REVIEW™ SERIES
Cardiac Problems
Respiratory Problems
Gastrointestinal Problems
Neurologic Problems

Nursing86 DRUG HANDBOOK™

Assessing Normal and Abnormal Breath Sounds

Breath sounds are produced by air moving through the tracheobron-
choalveolar system. Normal breath sounds are labeled *bronchial*, *bron-
chovesicular*, and *vesicular*. They're described according to location,
ratio of inspiration to expiration, intensity, and pitch.

Abnormal (adventitious) breath sounds occur when air passes either
through narrowed airways or through moisture, or when the membranes
lining the chest cavity and the lungs become inflamed. These sounds
include *rales*, *rhonchi*, *wheezes*, and *pleural friction rub*. You may hear
them superimposed over normal breath sounds.

Use this chart as a guide to assess both normal and abnormal breath
sounds. Document your findings.

TYPE/LOCATION	RATIO	DESCRIPTION
NORMAL BREATH SOUNDS		
Bronchial Over trachea	I 2:3 E	Loud, high-pitched, and hollow, harsh, or coarse
Bronchovesicular Anteriorly, near the mainstem bronchi in the first and second intercostal spaces; posteriorly, between the scapulae	I 1:1 E	Soft, breezy, and pitched about two notes lower than bronchial sounds
Vesicular In most of the lungs' peripheral parts (cannot be heard over the presternum or the scapulae)	I 3:1 E	Soft, swishy, breezy, and about two notes lower than broncho-vesicular sounds

Continued

RESPIRATORY CARE

Assessing Normal and Abnormal Breath Sounds
Continued

TYPE/LOCATION	CAUSE	DESCRIPTION
ABNORMAL BREATH SOUNDS		
Rales Anywhere. Heard in lung bases first with pulmonary edema, usually during inspiratory phase	Air passing through moisture, especially in the small airways and alveoli	Light crackling, popping, nonmusical; can be further classified by pitch: high, medium, or low
Rhonchi In larger airways, usually during expiratory phase	Fluid or secretions in the large airways or narrowing of large airways	Coarse rattling, usually louder and lower-pitched than rales; can be described as sonorous, bubbling, moaning, musical, sibilant, and rumbly
Wheezes Anywhere. Occurs during expiration	Narrowed airways	Creaking, groaning; always high-pitched, musical squeaks
Pleural friction rub Anterolateral lung field, on both inspiration and expiration (with the patient in an upright position)	Inflamed parietal and visceral pleural linings rubbing together	Superficial squeaking or grating

The Correct Percussion Sequence

Organize the percussion sequence so you move from more resonant body regions to less resonant ones. (You can perceive a change from resonance to dullness more easily than a change from dullness to resonance.) For example, when percussing to identify the lower border of liver dullness, start over the tympanic regions of the abdomen and then move up toward the dull area over the liver. To identify the liver's upper dullness border, begin over the lungs and percuss downward.

Identifying Percussion Sounds

Use this chart to help identify the sounds you may hear when percussing your patient's chest. Be sure to document your findings.

SOUND/PITCH	INTENSITY/QUALITY	INDICATION
Flatness High	Soft Extreme dullness	*Normal:* sternum; *abnormal:* atelectatic lung
Dullness Medium	Medium Thudlike	*Normal:* liver area, cardiac area, diaphragm; *abnormal:* pleural effusion
Resonance Low	Moderate to loud Hollow	*Normal:* lung
Hyperresonance Lower than resonance	Very loud Booming	*Abnormal:* emphysematous lung or pneumothorax
Tympany High	Loud Musical, drumlike	*Normal:* stomach area; *abnormal:* air-distended abdomen

Respiratory Acidosis

Alveolar hypoventilation causes respiratory retention of CO_2, leading to carbonic acid excess and a decreased pH. Arterial $PaCO_2$ above 45 mm Hg and pH below 7.35 characterize respiratory acidosis.

PREDISPOSING FACTORS

- Airway obstruction
- Chest-wall injury
- Neuromuscular disease
- Drug overdose (CNS depression)
- Adult respiratory distress syndrome
- Pneumothorax
- Pneumonia
- Pulmonary edema

SIGNS AND SYMPTOMS

- Tachycardia
- Shallow, slow respirations
- Dyspnea
- Dysrhythmias
- Cyanosis
- Diaphoresis
- Lethargy
- Confusion
- $PaCO_2 > 45$; pH < 7.35; but HCO_3^- 22 to 26 (normal)

COMPENSATION

- In the presence of *increased* $PaCO_2$, the kidneys compensate by excreting hydrogen ions and reabsorbing HCO_3^- to bring pH back to normal.

INTERVENTIONS

- Give O_2 (low concentrations in patients with chronic obstructive pulmonary disease).
- Give intravenous fluids.
- Give inhaled and/or intravenous bronchodilators.
- Start mechanical ventilation if hypoventilation can't be corrected immediately.
- Monitor ABGs and electrolytes.

Respiratory Alkalosis

Alveolar hyperventilation causes excess exhalation of CO_2, leading to carbonic acid deficit and an elevated pH. Arterial $PaCO_2$ below 35 mm Hg and pH above 7.45 characterize respiratory alkalosis.

PREDISPOSING FACTORS

- Extreme anxiety
- CNS injury to respiratory center
- Fever
- Overventilation during mechanical ventilation
- Pulmonary embolism
- Congestive heart failure
- Salicylate intoxication (early)

SIGNS AND SYMPTOMS

- Tachycardia
- Deep, rapid breathing
- Light-headedness
- Numbness and tingling or arm and leg paresthesias
- Carpopedal spasm
- Tetany
- $PaCO_2 < 35$; pH > 7.45; but HCO_3^- 22 to 26 (normal)

COMPENSATION

- In the presence of *decreased* $PaCO_2$, the kidneys compensate by retaining hydrogen ions and *not* reabsorbing HCO_3^- to bring pH back to normal.

INTERVENTIONS

- Have the patient breathe into a paper bag. (Rebreathing his CO_2 increases his $PaCO_2$.)
- Administer sedatives and give calm, reassuring support. (Hyperventilation is often triggered by "anxiety attacks.")
- Perform gastric lavage if salicylate overdose caused the alkalosis.
- Monitor ABGs and electrolytes.

Metabolic Acidosis

Metabolic acidosis is a state of *excess* acid accumulation and *deficient* bicarbonate (base) in the blood, resulting from conditions that cause:
- excessive fat metabolism in the absence of carbohydrates
- anaerobic metabolism
- underexcretion of metabolized acids or inability to conserve base
- loss of sodium bicarbonate from the intestines.

Arterial pH level is below 7.35; HCO_3^- is below 22 mEq/liter.

PREDISPOSING FACTORS

- Diabetic Ketoacidosis
- Addison's disease
- Renal failure
- Starvation
- Ethanol intoxication
- Tissue hypoxia
- Diarrhea
- Intestinal malabsorption
- Salicylate poisoning
- Low-carbohydrate, high-fat diet

SIGNS AND SYMPTOMS

- Headache and lethargy
- Central nervous system depression that may progress to coma
- Cardiac dysrhythmias
- Nausea and vomiting
- Anorexia
- Dehydration
- Kussmaul's respirations (a sign that respiratory compensation's beginning)

COMPENSATION

In the presence of low HCO_3^-, the respiratory system compensates with *hyperventilation* to *decrease* H_2CO_3 (as reflected in PCO_2) and to bring pH to normal by adjusting the ratio of HCO_3^- to H_2CO_3 to 20:1 (normal).

INTERVENTIONS

- Give the patient sodium bicarbonate I.V.
- Evaluate and correct his electrolyte imbalances.
- Observe precautions to prevent seizures.
- Monitor his vital signs and fluid balance.
- Treat the underlying cause, as ordered.

RESPIRATORY CARE

Metabolic Alkalosis

In contrast to metabolic acidosis, metabolic alkalosis is a state of *decreased* acid and *increased* bicarbonate (base) in the blood, resulting from conditions that cause:
- severe acid loss
- decreased serum potassium and chloride
- excessive bicarbonate intake.

Arterial pH level is above 7.45; HCO_3^- is above 29 mEq/liter.

PREDISPOSING FACTORS

- Vomiting
- GI suctioning
- Diuretic therapy
- Corticosteroid therapy
- Cushing's syndrome
- Excessive bicarbonate intake
- Hypokalemia
- Hypercalcemia

SIGNS AND SYMPTOMS

- Neuromuscular irritability
- Tetany
- Twitching
- Seizures
- Central nervous system depression that may progress to coma
- Cardiac dysrhythmias
- Nausea and vomiting
- Hypoventilation (a sign that respiratory compensation's beginning)

COMPENSATION

In the presence of high HCO_3^-, the respiratory system compensates with *hypoventilation* to *increase* H_2CO_3 (as reflected in PCO_2) and to bring pH to normal by adjusting the ratio of HCO_3^- to H_2CO_3 to 20:1 (normal).

INTERVENTIONS

- Give the patient normal saline solution and potassium I.V.
- Evaluate and correct his electrolyte imbalances.
- If his alkalosis is severe, give ammonium chloride I.V.
- Observe precautions to prevent seizures.
- Monitor his vital signs and fluid balance.
- Discontinue diuretics, if previously given.
- Treat the underlying cause, as ordered.

Assessing Emergency Respiratory Situations

CONDITION/NURSING ASSESSMENT	NURSING INTERVENTION
Acute respiratory arrest • No respiratory movement • No air felt over mouth and nose	• Position airway, using the head-tilt or jaw-thrust method. • Start mouth-to-mouth resuscitation immediately. • Once you've accomplished ventilation, continue until no longer needed. • Use endotracheal intubation and manual (or mechanical) ventilation, as ordered, for long-term support.
Complete airway obstruction • No respiratory movement • No air felt over mouth and nose • If conscious, patient attempts to speak but fails, and typically reaches for his throat	• Give four rapid blows between the scapulae, followed by the abdominal thrust or the midchest compression, as is done in external cardiac massage. • If airway remains obstructed, manual clearing may locate and remove obstruction. • Anticipate cricothyrotomy or tracheotomy if other attempts fail. Perform cricothyrotomy only in life-threatening emergency when a doctor is unavailable. Usually a doctor performs a tracheotomy in the operating room.
Partial airway obstruction • Increased respiratory effort • Noisy respirations • Use of accessory muscles, including abdominals, sternocleidomastoid, and internal intercostals • Possible intercostal retractions along with nasal flaring	• Administer back blows in succession. (This condition is unlikely to be relieved by an abdominal thrust or by chest compression.) • Administer oxygen until direct laryngoscopy becomes available.

Managing a Patient with Pulmonary Edema

STAGE/SYMPTOMS	NURSING RESPONSIBILITIES
Initial • Persistent cough—patient feels "like a cold is coming on" • Slight dyspnea/orthopnea • Exercise intolerance • Restlessness • Anxiety • Crepitant rales may be heard over the dependent portion of the lungs • Diastolic gallop	• Check color and amount of expectoration. • Position patient for comfort. • Auscultate chest for rales and third heart sound. • Medicate as ordered. • Monitor apical and radial pulses for rate and rhythm. • Assist patient with all needs to conserve strength. • Provide emotional support.
Advanced • Acute shortness of breath • Respirations—rapid, noisy (audible wheeze, rales) • Cough more intense and productive of frothy, blood-tinged sputum • Cyanosis • Diaphoresis—skin cold and clammy • Tachycardia—dysrhythmias • Hypotension	• Institute emergency measures: — Give oxygen—preferably by high-concentration mask or IPPB. — Insert I.V. if not already done. — Aspirate nasopharynx p.r.n. — Give digitalis and morphine, as ordered. — Give potent diuretics, as ordered. — Insert Foley catheter. — Draw ABGs. — Attach cardiac monitor leads and observe EKG. — Prepare for phlebotomy, if necessary. — Have resuscitation equipment available.
Acute • Decreased level of consciousness • Ventricular dysrhythmias • Shock • Diminished breath sounds	• Give emotional support. • Be prepared for cardioversion of tachydysrhythmias. • Assist with intubation and mechanical ventilation. • Resuscitate if necessary.

Recognizing the Stages of ARDS

Many emergency conditions (for example, lung contusion, drug overdose, or near drowning) can cause ARDS—adult respiratory distress
syndrome. In turn, ARDS can lead to acute respiratory failure, itself an
emergency.

You probably know what ARDS is: noncardiogenic pulmonary edema.
But can you recognize ARDS when it's developing? Recognition of high-
risk patients is the key to early detection and successful treatment of
ARDS. This chart will help you recognize the six developmental stages
of ARDS and intervene appropriately.

STAGE/SIGNS AND SYMPTOMS	NURSING INTERVENTIONS
1. Inflamed and damaged alveo-lar-capillary membrane • Depend on underlying cause of ARDS	• Do a brief assessment. • Take the patient's vital signs. • Auscultate for abnormal breath sounds. • Prepare the patient for a chest X-ray. • Begin treatment of underlying cause to prevent further ARDS development.
2. Protein and water shift in the interstitial space • Tachypnea, dyspnea, and tachy-cardia	• Draw blood for ABGs. • Prepare the patient for oxygen therapy, intubation, and mechani-cal ventilation. • Begin fluid management, avoid-ing fluid overload.
3. Pulmonary edema • Increased tachypnea, dyspnea, and cyanosis • Hypoxemia (generally unrespon-sive to increased FIO_2) • Decreased pulmonary compli-ance • Rales and rhonchi	• Connect the patient to a me-chanical ventilator with a positive end-expiratory pressure (PEEP) setting and a high oxygen con-centration. • Watch for complications from ventilation therapy.

Continued

Recognizing the Stages of ARDS
Continued

STAGE/SIGNS AND SYMPTOMS	NURSING INTERVENTIONS
4. Collapsed alveoli and impaired gas exchange • Thick, frothy, sticky sputum • Marked hypoxemia with increased respiratory distress	• Anticipate that a Swan-Ganz catheter will be inserted to measure pulmonary capillary wedge pressure.
5. Decreased oxygen and carbon dioxide levels in the blood • Increased tachypnea • Hypoxemia • Hypocapnia	• Study ABGs, mixed venous blood gases, and pulmonary capillary wedge pressure to understand the relationship between PEEP, intrapulmonary shunt, and cardiac output. • Monitor the patient's vital signs and urine output (hydration).
6. Hypoxemia; metabolic acidosis • Decreased serum pH • Increased $PaCO_2$ level • Decreased PaO_2 level • Confusion • Decreased HCO_3^- level	• Watch for fluid restriction or overdiuresis that may cause hypovolemia, hypotension, and hypoperfusion. • Check for shock, coma, respiratory failure, and neurologic complications secondary to metabolic alterations and respiratory failure. • Reassure the patient and his family.

Guide to Artificial Airways

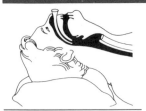 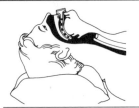

NASOPHARYNGEAL

Indications
- Airway obstruction, when oropharyngeal airway is contraindicated because of trauma to lower face or oral surgery
- Surgery, to maintain patent airway until patient recovers from anesthesia

Contraindications
- Nasal obstruction
- Predisposition to epistaxis

Advantages
- Inserted easily
- Tolerated better than oropharyngeal airway by conscious patients
- Allows for suctioning without displacing the patient's nasal turbinates

Disadvantages
- May cause severe epistaxis if inserted too forcefully
- Kinks and clogs easily, obstructing airway
- May cause pressure necrosis of nasal mucosa
- May cause air passage obstruction, if artificial airway is too large

OROPHARYNGEAL

Indications
- Airway obstruction, when nasopharyngeal airway is contraindicated because of nasal obstruction or predisposition to epistaxis
- Short-term intubation

Contraindications
- Trauma to lower face
- Before, during, or after oral surgery

Advantages
- Inserted easily
- Holds tongue away from pharynx
- Tolerated well by patients

Disadvantages
- Dislodged easily
- May stimulate gag reflex
- May cause obstruction if airway size is incorrect

Continued

Guide to Artificial Airways
Continued

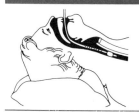 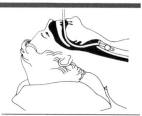

ORAL ESOPHAGEAL

Indications
• Airway obstruction, when all other efforts to maintain an open airway have failed. (Used primarily in emergency departments or by trained paramedics.)
Contraindications
• Trauma to lower face
• Before, during, or after oral surgery
Advantages
• Inserted quickly and easily
• Prevents aspiration of stomach contents while tube is in place
Disadvantages
• May cause pharyngeal trauma during insertion
• May be accidentally inserted into trachea
• May cause gastric distention and impair ventilation if cuff is improperly inflated
• Allows possible aspiration of stomach contents during tube removal

ORAL ENDOTRACHEAL

Indications
• Cardiopulmonary resuscitation or other airway obstruction, when all other efforts to maintain an airway have failed, and when patient has nasal obstruction or predisposition to epistaxis
• Mechanical ventilation, when patient has nasal obstruction or predisposition to epistaxis
• Short-term intubation
Contraindications
• Trauma to lower face
• Before, during, or after oral surgery
• Long-term intubation
Advantages
• Inserted quickly and easily
• Causes less intubation trauma than nasal endotracheal airway
• Permits use of a large diameter tube

Continued

Guide to Artificial Airways
Continued

ORAL ENDOTRACHEAL
Continued

• Eliminates danger of introducing infection or blood from nasal fossae into trachea
• Involves less tissue destruction than with trach tube
• Prevents aspiration of stomach contents, if cuff is inflated

Disadvantages
• May damage teeth or lacerate lips, mouth, pharyngeal mucosa, or larynx during insertion
• May cause aspiration of blood or vomitus during insertion
• Activates gag reflex in conscious patients
• Kinks and clogs easily, obstructing airway
• Interferes with cough reflex
• Prevents patient from talking, if cuff is inflated
• May be bitten or chewed
• May cause pressure necrosis
• May stimulate retching, which can lead to gastric distention
• May cause laryngeal edema, apnea secondary to reflexive breath holding, bronchospasms, or infection
• May cause tracheal damage

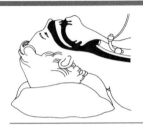

TRACHEOSTOMY

Indications
• Complete upper airway obstruction, when endotracheal intubation is impossible
• Long-term intubation

Contraindications
• Intubation of infants
• Whenever patient is highly susceptible to infection; for example, when he's receiving an immunosuppressant drug
• Short-term intubation

Advantages
• Suctioned more easily than endotracheal tube
• Decreases dead air space in respiratory system more than other airways do
• Permits patient to swallow and eat

Continued

Guide to Artificial Airways
Continued

TRACHEOSTOMY
Continued

• Feels more comfortable than other tubes
• Prevents aspiration of stomach contents, if cuff is inflated
Disadvantages
• Requires surgery to insert
• Can't be used for infants
• May cause laceration or pressure necrosis of trachea, especially in children

• May cause tracheoesophageal fistula
• Increases risk of tracheal and stomal inflammation
• Entails major risk of infection
• Increases risk of mucous plugs
• Prevents patient from talking, if cuff is inflated

Choosing the Correct Size Tube

Is the doctor about to perform a tracheotomy or intubate your patient? Then, observe the following important guidelines:
• Always examine the patient *before* you consider tubing size. Look for unusual features or conditions that may affect the size of his nasal or oral passage: for example, overdeveloped neck muscles; a relatively small nose; signs of tracheal or epiglottal edema.
• When you know the range of recommended sizes for your particular patient, select the tube with the largest internal diameter to permit better gas flow.
• The patient who undergoes a tracheotomy may need an adjustment in tube size once postopera-

tive edema diminishes. Watch for an enlargement in stoma size, which indicates the swelling has gone down. Notify the doctor.
• Don't expect to find cuffs on tracheostomy and endotracheal tubes under size 5 or 5.5 (generally used to intubate children). In a child, cuff pressure is hard to regulate and may cause severe damage.
• If the doctor specifies a Shiley tracheostomy tube, remember you can only get it in even sizes: 4, 6, 8, or 10.
• Suppose you know the internal diameter of an endotracheal tube and want the French size. To get it, multiply the diameter by 4.

Guide to Drugs Used During Intubation

PANCURONIUM BROMIDE

Drug
Pavulon*

Indications and dosages
To induce skeletal muscle relaxation for intubation and to facilitate mechanical ventilation:
Adults and children: Initially 0.06 to 0.1 mg per kg I.V. Additional doses at 30- to 60-minute intervals.

Side effects
Tachycardia, increased blood pressure, burning sensation at injection site, skin rash, sweating, excessive salivation.

Nursing considerations
• Monitor patient's vital signs and keep his airway clear until he's completely recovered from the effects of this drug.
• Don't give drug without doctor's direct supervision; never leave patient unattended.
• Patient must be ventilated until drug's effect wears off.
• Patient must have nasogastric tube.
• Instill artificial tears and patch patient's eyes.

• Change patient's position frequently.
• Refrigerate medication.
• Don't mix with barbiturate solutions.
• Being totally paralyzed by this drug will no doubt terrify your patient. The doctor may give him medication to relax him.
• Do not store in plastic containers or syringes, although plastic syringes may be used for administration.
• Allow succinylcholine effects to subside before giving pancuronium.

SUCCINYLCHOLINE CHLORIDE

Drug
Anectine*, Anectine Flo-Pack*, Quelicin*, Sucostrin, Sux-Cert

Indications and dosages
To induce skeletal muscle relaxation for intubation and to facilitate mechanical ventilation:
Adults: 40 to 100 mg I.V.
Infants and children:
1 to 2 mg/kg I.V. For I.M. administration:

*Available in the United States and Canada.
**Available only in Canada.

Continued

Guide to Drugs Used During Intubation
Continued

SUCCINYLCHOLINE
CHLORIDE
Continued

Adults, infants, and children: 2.5 mg/kg. Max. dose: 150 mg
Side effects
Bradycardia, tachycardia, blood pressure changes, dysrhythmias, cardiac arrest, increased intraocular pressure, apnea, hyperthermia, myoglobinemia, excessive salivation.
Nursing considerations
• Observe first six precautions listed for pancuronium bromide.
• Being totally paralyzed by this drug will terrify your patient.
• Store in refrigerator; use only fresh solutions.
• Don't mix with barbiturates.
• Give test dose of 10 mg I.V. to check for sensitivity and recovery time.
• Inject deep into deltoid muscle when giving I.M.
• Repeated or continued infusions of succinylcholine alone not advised; may cause reduced response or prolonged apnea.

TUBOCURARINE
CHLORIDE

Drug
Tubarine*
Indications and dosages
To induce skeletal muscle relaxation for intubation and to facilitate mechanical ventilation:
Adults: 40 to 60 units I.V. or 0.1 to 0.3 mg/kg I.M. or I.V.
Side effects
Hypotension, circulatory or respiratory depression, increased secretions, decreased GI motility, hypersensitivity. Rapid I.V. injection may cause bronchospasm.
Nursing considerations
• Observe first six precautions listed for pancuronium bromide.
• Being totally paralyzed by this drug will terrify your patient. To relax him, the doctor will probably order morphine.
• Use only fresh solutions; don't use solution that's discolored.
• Don't mix with barbiturate solutions.
• Inject deep into deltoid muscle when giving I.M.

Continued

Guide to Drugs Used During Intubation
Continued

TUBOCURARINE
CHLORIDE
Continued

• Do not give without direct supervision of doctor.
• Monitor respirations every 5 to 15 minutes and before each I.V.-repeated dose. Have emergency resuscitation equipment and oxygen at bedside.
• Avoid extravasation.
• Do not infuse drug through plastic tubing. Do not store in plastic syringe.
• Drug should not be withdrawn abruptly.

DIAZEPAM

Drug
D-Tran**, E-Pam**, Paxel**, Valium*
Indications and dosages
To relieve anxiety prior to intubation and to facilitate mechanical ventilation:

Adults: 2 to 20 mg every 3 to 4 hours I.M. or I.V., depending on patient's response.
Children over age 1 month: 1 to 2 mg every 3 to 4 hours I.M. or I.V.
Side effects
Bradycardia, hypotension, tachycardia, edema, cardiovascular collapse, skin rash, laryngospasm. With I.M. injection, possible local irritation and pain at injection site. With rapid I.V. injection, cardiac arrest.
Nursing considerations
• Monitor vital signs and keep airway free of secretions.
• Don't mix or dilute parenteral form with other I.V. fluids.
• Inject slowly when giving I.V., allowing at least 1 minute per 5 mg.
• Use extreme care when administering drug to elderly or debilitated patients.
• Inject deep into large muscle mass when giving I.M.

*Available in the United States and Canada.
**Available only in Canada.

Securing an Endotracheal Tube: Three Methods

Before taping the tube in place, make sure the patient's face is clean, dry, and free of beard stubble. If possible, suction his mouth and dry off the tube just before taping. After taping, always check for bilateral breath sounds to ensure the tube hasn't been displaced by manipulation.

1. Cut two 2″ (5-cm) strips and two 15″ (38-cm) strips of 1″ cloth adhesive tape. Then, cut a 13″ (33-cm) slit in one end of each 15″ strip (see illustration below).

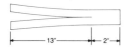

Apply benzoin to the patient's cheeks.* Place the 2″ strips on his cheeks, creating a new surface on which to anchor the tape securing the endotracheal tube. *When frequent retaping is necessary, this helps preserve the patient's skin's integrity.* If the patient's skin is excoriated or at risk, you can use OP-Site to protect the skin.

Apply benzoin to the tape on the patient's face and to the part of the tube where you will be applying the tape.

On the side of the mouth where the tube will be anchored, place the unslit end of a 15″ strip of tape on top of the tape on the patient's cheek. Just before taping, check the reference mark on the tube to ensure correct placement.

Wrap the top half of the tape around the tube twice, pulling the tape as tightly as possible. Then, directing the tape over the patient's upper lip, place the end of the tape on the patient's other cheek. Cut off any excess tape.

Use the lower half of the tape to secure an oral airway, if necessary (see illustration below). Or, twist the lower half of the tape around the tube twice and attach it

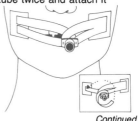

Continued

Securing an Endotracheal Tube: Three Methods
Continued

to the original cheek (see illustration below). *Taping in opposite directions places equal traction on the tube.*

If you've taped in an oral airway or are concerned about tube stability, apply the other 15″ strip of tape in the same manner as the first, starting on the other side of the patient's face. If the tape around the tube is too bulky, use only the upper part of the tape and cut off the lower part. If copious oral secretions are present, seal the tape by cutting a 1″ (2.5-cm) piece of paper tape, coating it with benzoin, and placing the paper tape over the adhesive tape.

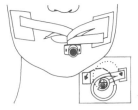

2. Cut one piece of 1″ cloth adhesive tape long enough to wrap around the patient's

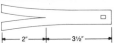

head and overlap in front. Then, cut an 8″ (20-cm) piece of tape and center it on the longer piece, sticky sides together. Next, cut a 5″ (12.5-cm) slit in each end (see illustration above).

Apply benzoin to the patient's cheeks and under his nose.†

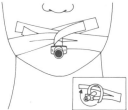

Place the top half of one end of the tape under the patient's nose and wrap the lower half around the endotracheal tube. Place the lower half of the other end of the tape under the patient's nose and wrap the top half around the tube (see illustration above).

Continued

Securing an Endotracheal Tube: Three Methods
Continued

3. Cut a tracheostomy tie in two pieces (one a few inches longer than the other), and cut two 6" (15-cm) pieces of 1" cloth adhesive tape. Then, cut a 2" slit in one end of both pieces of tape. Fold the other end of the tape so the sticky sides are together and cut a small hole in it (see illustration below).

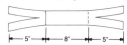

|← 5″ →|← 8″ →|← 5″ →|

Apply benzoin to the part of the endotracheal tube that will be taped.

Wrap the slit ends of each piece of tape around the tube—one piece on each side. To secure the tape, overlap it.

Apply the free ends of the tape to both sides of the patient's face. Then, insert the tracheostomy ties through the holes on the ends of the tape

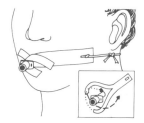

and knot the ties (see illustration above).

Bring the longer tie behind the patient's neck and tie it to the shorter tie at one side of his neck. *Knotting the ties on the side prevents the patient from lying on the knot and getting a pressure sore.*

---

†Don't spray benzoin directly on the patient's face because its vapors can be irritating if inhaled and can be harmful to the eyes.

Problems with Artificial Airways: How to Correct Them

PROBLEM	SUSPECT IT WHEN

Tracheoesophageal fistula

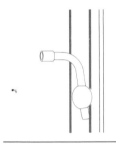

- You detect a significant air leak through the stoma or nose and mouth even though cuff is up.
- You suction the patient's airway and observe food or liquid in the aspirate.
- The patient belches frequently.
- The patient coughs every time he swallows.
- You get positive results from a methylene blue test.

Underinflated cuff

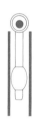

- You detect a significant air leak through the stoma, nose, or mouth. The ventilator shows a decrease in the patient's expired volume.

TO TREAT THE PATIENT	TO AVOID THE COMPLICATION
• Don't feed the patient until the extent of the fistula is determined. • Suction his trachea through the tube only. • Administer prophylactic antibiotics for aspiration pneumonia on doctor's orders. • The doctor may remove the tube and order hyperalimentation.	• Use a low-pressure cuff and the minimal leak technique. • Exercise meticulous cuff care.
• Inflate the cuff to the proper size. Make sure you use the minimal leak technique.	• Follow the manufacturer's recommendations on cuff volume as an initial guide, but then use the minimal leak technique. • Measure cuff pressure immediately after inflation, and routinely check pressure.

Continued

RESPIRATORY CARE

Problems with Artificial Airways: How to Correct Them
Continued

PROBLEM	SUSPECT IT WHEN

Ruptured cuff

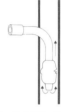

* You detect a significant air leak through the stoma, nose, or mouth.
* No pressure registers on a manometer check.
* The ventilator shows a decrease in the patient's expired volume.
* The ventilator's low-pressure alarm sounds.

Herniated cuff blocking the end of the tube

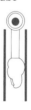

* You feel an obstruction in the tube when you're suctioning.
* Low-pressure alarm sounds on patient's ventilator.
* Patient experiences moderate difficulty on inhalation. Exhalation may be completely blocked.

TO TREAT THE PATIENT	TO AVOID THE COMPLICATION
• Notify the doctor, and prepare to change the tube.	• Check the cuff's symmetry by inflating it before insertion. • Avoid accidentally pulling the cuff into the suction catheter when you're performing nasotracheal suctioning.
• Replace the tube immediately. Have a replacement on hand.	• Check the cuff for symmetrical inflation *before* you insert the tube. • Avoid overinflation of the cuff.

Continued

Problems with Artificial Airways: How to Correct Them
Continued

PROBLEM	SUSPECT IT WHEN
Carina or wall of trachea obstructs tube lumen 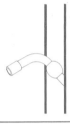	• You have difficulty forcing air into the tube with a hand ventilator. • You feel an obstruction in the tube when you're suctioning. • You note that the patient's blood gas measurement shows a decrease in PO_2. • The ventilator's pressure alarm sounds. • The patient seems anxious and agitated (air hunger).
Secretions obstruct tube lumen 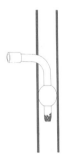	• You feel an obstruction in the tube when suctioning.

TO TREAT THE PATIENT	TO AVOID THE COMPLICATION
• Deflate cuff and reposition tube.	• Make sure you select the proper-sized tube. • Tape the tubing securely. • Tie the trach ties snugly.
• Move suction catheter to one side to pass obstruction. • Instill saline, hyperinflate the patient's lungs, and suction him with a correct-sized catheter. • The doctor may want to change the tube, order bronchodilator drugs, or give the patient I.V. therapy. • Humidify the patient's airway. • Perform meticulous trach care. • Perform postural drainage, percussion, and vibration.	• Use humidified oxygen to keep secretions thin. • The doctor may order cooled or heated aerosol treatments periodically. He may also order forced fluids or I.V. therapy.

Continued

Problems with Artificial Airways: How to Correct Them

Continued

PROBLEM	SUSPECT IT WHEN
For endotracheal tubes only	

| *Kinked tube* 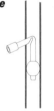 | • You feel an obstruction in the tube when suctioning.
• The patient's blood gas measurement shows a decrease in PO_2.
• The ventilator's pressure alarm sounds. |

| *Tube in right main bronchus* 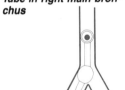 | • You hear few, if any, breath sounds in the left lung.
• You observe asymmetrical chest expansion. |

Warning: Accidental Extubation

Any number of events may lead to endotracheal extubation. For example, a confused or disoriented patient may pull out the tube; saliva may loosen the tape anchoring the tube; or the tape may not stick well to a diaphoretic patient's skin.

Nursing interventions
• Remove any portion of the tube that's still in place.

Continued

TO TREAT THE PATIENT	TO AVOID THE COMPLICATION
• Working quickly, deflate the cuff. Then, insert the stylet to straighten out the tubing. • Withdraw the tube, and cut it to the correct length, if needed. Tape securely.	• Slacken the tension on the ventilator and oxygen tubing so it doesn't pull on the endotracheal tube. • Always make sure the endotracheal tube's the proper size before you insert it. • Tape the endotracheal tube securely in place.
• Withdraw the endotracheal tube slightly. Then, carefully reposition it and recheck breath sounds.	• Check the X-ray for proper placement immediately after insertion. • Trim off any excess tubing. • Tape the tube securely to prevent slipping.

Warning: Accidental Extubation
Continued

• Ventilate the patient using mouth-to-mouth resuscitation or an Ambu (or anesthesia) bag.
• Send someone to notify the doctor to reintubate the patient.
• Restrain the patient if he has purposely extubated himself, to prevent him from doing it again.
• Each time the patient is repositioned, check the tape holding the reinserted tube.
• To make the tube secure, anchor tape from the nape of his neck to and around the tube.

Understanding Mechanical Ventilation Techniques

If your patient is hypoxemic or can't breathe spontaneously, he'll need supplemental oxygen, mechanical ventilation, or both. The doctor orders the therapy, of course. But understanding how it works will help you reinforce your patient's breathing efforts, monitor the therapy's effectiveness, and do more effective patient teaching.

Here's a chart that explains some commonly used ventilation and supplemental oxygen techniques and gives you nursing tips for administering them. Remember, your patient's recovery—and maybe his life—depend on the equipment's smooth functioning. To ensure this, watch for equipment malfunctions and observe your patient for signs and symptoms of oxygen toxicity and carbon dioxide retention. Monitor his vital signs frequently.

CONTINUOUS POSITIVE AIRWAY PRESSURE (C.P.A.P.)

Uses
• Improves arterial oxygenation from ventilation-perfusion imbalances
• Opens alveoli and improves functional residual capacity
• Supplements oxygen therapy for patients not needing mechanical ventilation
• Helps treat adult respiratory distress syndrome (ARDS), acute respiratory failure (ARF), and reduced surfactant production

Mechanism
• The patient breathes while oxygen is delivered through an endotracheal tube or tight-fitting mask (with narrow opening to retard expiration) at constant pressure throughout the respiratory cycle.

Nursing Considerations
• Make sure the patient is alert and able to communicate.
• Insert an endotracheal tube or apply a mask.
• Insert a nasogastric tube to decompress the stomach and to avoid distention and vomiting.
• Monitor the amount of positive pressure with an aneroid manometer.
• Watch for decreased cardiac output from high CPAP levels.
• Watch for fatigue and carbon dioxide retention from increased work of breathing.

Continued

Understanding Mechanical Ventilation Techniques
Continued

POSITIVE END-EXPIRATORY PRESSURE (P.E.E.P.)

Uses
• Keeps airways and alveoli from collapsing
• Helps stabilize a flail chest and treat ARDS and ARF
• Increases functional residual capacity

Mechanism
• The ventilator keeps positive pressure in alveoli and airways through end expiration, reinflating collapsed alveoli.
• Low oxygen concentrations increase arterial oxygen pressure.

Nursing considerations
• Prepare chest tubes, Pleurevac, and thoracotomy tray in case tension pneumothorax develops.
• Watch for decreased cardiac output caused by increased intrathoracic pressure and low venous return.
• Watch for increased intracranial pressure.

INTERMITTENT MANDATORY VENTILATION (I.M.V.)

Uses
• Lets the patient assist ventilation with his own breathing
• Weans him from the ventilator
• Reduces the chance of pneumothorax and decreased cardiac output

Mechanism
• The ventilator mandatorily delivers a preset number of breaths per minute.
• The patient breathes on his own between preset mandatory breaths, inspiring ventilator's set percentage of oxygen.

Nursing considerations
• Take the patient's ABGs to monitor therapy.
• Reduce the frequency of assisted breaths as the patient weans himself from the ventilator.
• Reassure the patient about fears of leaving the ventilator.

Continued

Understanding Mechanical Ventilation Techniques
Continued

HIGH-FREQUENCY VENTILATION (H.F.V.)

Uses
● Supplements PEEP and CPAP
● Ventilates a patient under anesthesia for rigid bronchoscopy and direct laryngoscopy
● Helps treat bronchopleural fistulae and adult and infant respiratory distress syndromes
● Maintains cardiac output and improves gas exchange during mechanical ventilation

Mechanism
● The ventilator gives 60 to 3,000 breaths/minute (depending on the type of HFV) with low tidal volume, low airway pressure, and brief inspiratory time.

Nursing considerations
● Closely monitor vital signs.
● Adjust humidification infusion, as needed, to prevent secretions from becoming too viscous.

VOLUME-CYCLED VENTILATOR

Uses
● Artificially controls or assists respiration or encourages spontaneous breathing, while guaranteeing minimum ventilation support
● Corrects serious gas exchange abnormalities in hypoxemia, hypercapnia, and labored breathing

Mechanism
● The ventilator delivers preset tidal volume and rate to a patient not breathing on his own (control).
● If the patient breathes slightly on his own, the ventilator senses his breath, then delivers full tidal volume (assist).

Nursing considerations
● Place the patient in a semi-Fowler position to encourage lung expansion.
● Monitor the patient's ABGs and blood pressure to assess oxygen and carbon dioxide levels, ventilation effectiveness, and oxygen toxicity.
● Administer several deep breaths hourly to prevent alveolar collapse and to stimulate coughing.
● Check for atelectasis.
● Beware of anxiety in the patient. He may need sedation.

Coping with Mechanical Ventilation Complications

BAROTRAUMA

Takes the form of pneumo-thorax, subcutaneous emphysema, or mediastinal emphysema. Usually caused when volume and pressure settings are too high or during positive end-expiratory pressure (PEEP) administration.

Signs and symptoms
Sudden cyanosis, drop in blood pressure, and decrease in lung compliance; increased anxiety. With pneumothorax, patient may have absent or diminished breath sounds over affected lung segment; acute pain on affected side, and trachea deviated away from pneumothorax. With subcutaneous emphysema, patient may have crepitus of face, abdomen, and extremities. With mediastinal emphysema, patient shows signs of reduced cardiac output and of crepitus over heart area.

Treatment
● Call doctor immediately; he may insert chest tubes.

Prevention
● Avoid high-pressure settings for high-risk patients.

ATELECTASIS

Caused by insufficient deep breathing, pneumothorax, secretion retention, or a combination of these.

Signs and symptoms
Transient fine crackles; diminished breath sounds over affected lung segment; bronchial sounds over peripheral lung fields; decreased compliance; possible change in arterial blood gas (ABG) values.

Treatment
● Turn patient frequently.
● Suction and hyperinflate patient's lungs periodically.
● Use intermittent sighing.
● Perform chest physiotherapy, as ordered.
● Doctor may order bronchoscopy.

Prevention
● Change patient's position every 1 to 2 hours.
● Give chest physiotherapy, and maintain good pulmonary hygiene.
● Doctor may order PEEP.
● Suction the patient, as needed.
● Remember to sigh patient.
● Monitor the patient closely.

Continued

Coping with Mechanical Ventilation Complications
Continued

CARDIOVASCULAR IMPAIRMENT

Caused when positive intrathoracic pressure reduces venous return to heart's right side and compresses pulmonary blood circulation.

Signs and symptoms
Decreased blood pressure and cardiac output; possible decreased urinary output; increased central venous pressure and pulmonary artery pressure; increased heart rate.

Treatment
• Doctor may reduce intrathoracic pressure by decreasing PEEP, inspiratory flow rate, or tidal volume.
• Doctor may order increased I.V. fluids or administration of plasma expanders such as albumin or colloidal substances.

Prevention
• Monitor PaO_2 closely. It should not fall below 70 mm Hg.
• Use PEEP only when necessary.
• Shorten inspiration time to less than one-half expiration time.
• Maintain adequate blood volume.

GASTROINTESTINAL COMPLICATIONS

Caused by stress or swallowing air. Such complications include GI bleeding, gastric distention, paralytic ileus, and stress ulcer.

Signs and symptoms
Abdominal distention; steady decrease in hemoglobin and hematocrit measurement; positive hematest results on nasogastric drainage and stool; tarry stool.

Treatment
• As ordered, insert nasogastric tube for drainage.
• Replace lost blood.
• Use nasogastric tube to give antacids or other medication to decrease acid production.

Prevention
• Avoid giving excessive positive pressure.
• Reduce patient's psychological stress.
• Give antacids and other medications to reduce acid production, as ordered.

Continued

Coping with Mechanical Ventilation Complications
Continued

ACID-BASE AND FLUID AND ELECTROLYTE IMBALANCE

Caused by positive water balance created by secretion of antidiuretic hormone (ADH). Also caused by reduced insensible losses from respiratory tract.

Signs and symptoms
Probable change in blood gas measurements; decreased vital capacity; weight gain; ankle edema; moist rales in lungs' lower lobes; pulmonary edema confirmed by X-ray.

Treatment
• Doctor may restrict fluid intake and order diuretics.
• Treat the patient for congestive heart failure (CHF), as ordered.
• Apply rotating tourniquets to control pulmonary edema, as ordered.
• Correct acid-base imbalance, as ordered.
• Correct electrolyte imbalance, as ordered.

Prevention
• Periodically obtain blood samples for ABG and electrolyte measurements. Monitor patient for hyperventilation or hypoventilation.
• Monitor patient's fluid intake and output.
• Weigh patient daily.

TRACHEAL TRAUMA

Caused by constant pressure of cuffed endotracheal tube or nasal endotracheal tube on the patient's trachea.

Signs and symptoms
Decreased tidal volume from air leak; bleeding from trachea.

Treatment
• Depending on damage, the doctor may insert a new trach tube to change cuff's position and allow injured area to heal.
• Give meticulous cuff care, using minimal leak technique, until tube can be removed.

Prevention
• Give patient proper cuff care, using minimal leak technique when possible.
• Doctor should use endotracheal or trach tubes with soft cuffs.

Continued

Coping with Mechanical Ventilation Complications
Continued

RESPIRATORY INFECTION

Caused when upper airway is bypassed, eliminating body's natural defense mechanisms against infection. Also caused by poor aseptic technique.

Signs and symptoms
Elevated temperature and white blood cell count (WBC); increased amount of respiratory secretions, and change in their color and odor.

Treatment
• Notify doctor.
• Change patient's position frequently and perform chest physiotherapy.
• Use aseptic technique for trach care and for suctioning.
• Administer prescribed antibiotics.

Prevention
• Maintain good pulmonary hygiene by using aseptic technique and sterile equipment, changing ventilator tubing every 24 hours, and suctioning patient and hyperinflating his lungs as needed.
• Turn patient frequently.
• Perform chest physiotherapy.
• Filter all inspired gas.

OXYGEN TOXICITY

Caused by excessively high concentrations of oxygen (over 60%) administered over prolonged period (8 hours or more). May cause fibrotic tissue changes in lungs, possibly leading to death.

Signs and symptoms
Retrosternal pain; sore throat; nasal congestion; burning chest pain on inspiration; dry, hacking cough; dyspnea; decreased compliance; decreased PaO_2 on the same oxygen concentration; decreased vital capacity; and X-ray changes.

Treatment
• Monitor oxygen levels carefully. Report signs of oxygen toxicosis immediately.

Prevention
• Maintain good pulmonary hygiene so low oxygen concentrations are adequate.
• Reduce oxygen concentrations as soon as possible.
• Use PEEP to reduce oxygen concentration level, as ordered.

After Angiography: Caring for Your Patient

Pulmonary angiography is the radiographic examination of the pulmonary circulation following injection of a radiopaque iodine contrast agent through a catheter inserted into the pulmonary artery or one of its branches. Most commonly, this invasive technique is used to confirm symptomatic pulmonary emboli when scans prove nondiagnostic, especially in patients in whom anticoagulant therapy is contraindicated. It also provides accurate preoperative evaluation of patients with congenital heart disease. When a patient returns to your unit after angiography, make him as comfortable as possible. Also, be sure to watch him closely for complications, using these guidelines.

• Apply ice packs to the puncture site. Doing so helps control swelling, minimizes the risk of hemorrhage, and promotes patient comfort.

• Frequently check the pressure bandage over the puncture site. Keep the bandage dry and secure.

• If bleeding occurs, apply direct pressure to the puncture site. Have a co-worker notify the doctor.

• Observe the puncture site for any redness or swelling which may indicate a hematoma. If these symptoms are present, notify the doctor.

• Take vital signs, and perform a neurocheck every 15 minutes for at least an hour, until the patient's stable. Then, continue to take his vital signs and perform neurochecks frequently, as ordered.

• At least once every half hour, check below the puncture site for pulse, color, warmth, and movement.

• Immobilize the patient's affected arm or leg, for 4 to 6 hours to discourage bleeding.

• Make sure the patient gets at least 12 hours of complete bed rest, as ordered.

• Encourage your patient to drink plenty of fluids. Monitor his output carefully. Because contrast dye acts as a diuretic, your patient may become dehydrated.

• After the doctor has explained the results to your patient and his family, be available to answer any questions they may have.

• Document all observations in your patient's chart and in your notes. Notify the doctor of any complications immediately.

RESPIRATORY CARE

Ventilator Warning Signals: How to Respond

SIGNALS/PROBLEM	CAUSE
Pressure alarm sounds when delivery of preset volume requires higher pressures than pressure limit permits. • Airway obstruction	• Secretions • Kink in tubes • Endotracheal or trach tube out of position
• High resistance	• Secretions • Bronchospasm • Water from humidifier in ventilator tubing
• Decrease in compliance	• Pulmonary edema • Adult respiratory distress syndrome (ARDS) • Pneumothorax • Pneumonia

NURSING CONSIDERATIONS

• Suction the patient, instilling saline solution to loosen secretions.

• Straighten tubes and provide support for them.

• Reposition tube.

• Suction the secretions.
• Provide chest physiotherapy.

• Administer bronchodilators, as ordered.
• Decrease flow rate and tidal volume.

• Drain the water.
• Check to see if water temperature's higher than 96.8° F. (36° C.).

• Administer diuretics and restrict fluids, as ordered.

• Doctor will probably order continuous positive airway pressure (CPAP) or positive end-expiratory pressure (PEEP).

• Doctor will insert chest tubes.

• Administer antibiotics, as ordered.
• Give fluids, as ordered.
• Provide chest physiotherapy.

Continued

Ventilator Warning Signals: How to Respond
Continued

SIGNALS/PROBLEM	CAUSE
• Patient fighting ventilator	• Hypoxia
	• Fear, anxiety
	• Improvement in patient's condition
Spirometer alarm sounds when tidal volume is less than preset volume. • Leak or disconnection	• Loose connection in tubing, nebulizer, humidifier, endotracheal tube, or trach tube
	• Cuff insufficiently inflated

NURSING CONSIDERATIONS

• Inspect patient for symptoms of hypoxia, such as confusion, dyspnea, cyanosis, and tachycardia.
• Draw arterial blood to obtain arterial blood gas measurements. If ABG measurements indicate hypoxia, notify doctor so he can adjust the oxygen concentration order.
• Suction patient and hyperinflate his lungs, as needed.

• Ask patient if he feels he's getting enough air.
• To make sure the patient's not actually hypoxic, inspect him for hypoxia symptoms. If inspection indicates hypoxia, draw arterial blood for blood gas measurements.
• Try to calm patient. Give him writing materials so he can communicate. Give sedative or muscle relaxants, if ordered.

• Begin weaning when ordered by doctor.
• Adjust sensitivity setting, as needed.

• Carefully check each connection in system.
• Reconnect tubing if it's loose.
• Be sure humidifier or nebulizer lids fit tightly.
• Check to see that the spirometer's rubber seal fits tightly.

• Deflate cuff and inflate again. If cuff won't seal and patient's still not getting prescribed tidal volume, call the doctor. Use a hand-held resuscitator to ventilate patient's lungs until a new tube can be inserted.

Continued

RESPIRATORY CARE

Ventilator Warning Signals: How to Respond
Continued

SIGNALS/PROBLEM	CAUSE
• Defect in spirometer action	• Water or dirt in spirometer
	• Spirometer incorrectly attached
	• Defective spirometer
	• Tubing support arm leaning on dipstick, interfering with bellows movement
• Power interruption	• Faulty electrical connection
Oxygen light activates because of incorrect oxygen concentration • Oxygen not connected to ventilator	• Disconnection or failure to connect properly
• Dirty oxygen filter or dirty air intake filter	• Improper maintenance

NURSING CONSIDERATIONS

- Dry or clean the spirometer.

- Check the manufacturer's instructions.

- Check position of diaphragm on the spirometer's base.
- Check dump valve (black tube) fit on spirometer base.
- Replace the spirometer, if necessary.

- Readjust arm so that it clears the dipstick.
- Check circuit breaker.
- Check whether plug's firmly in wall outlet.

- Connect ventilator tubing to oxygen outlet.

- Remove filter, clean with warm, soapy water, and dry.

New Advances in Respiratory Monitoring—Oximetry

Until recently, you had to rely on arterial blood gas (ABG) measurements to sound the alarm when acute hypoxemia threatened your patient's life. But many hospitals now are using a new, improved version of an old procedure—oximetry—to provide continuous monitoring of arterial oxygenation in patients with cardiorespiratory disorders.

An oximeter monitors your patient's oxygen saturation continuously, so it rapidly (within 6 seconds) detects any trend in his oxygenation status—unlike ABGs, which you can measure only periodically. And because oximetry's a simple, noninvasive procedure, you don't need to be specially trained to do it. Here's how these devices work.

An *ear oximeter* measures a patient's arterial oxygen saturation by monitoring the transmission of two light waves through his earlobe's vascular bed. Light emitters and sensors are contained in an ear probe that you clip to your patient's earlobe. A heater in the ear probe's tip maintains the skin's surface temperature at 98.6° F. (37°C.), dilating the arterial vascular bed to enable more accurate readings. A cable conducts the ear probe's electrical signal to the oximeter, which calculates oxygen saturation and displays the values on a digital-readout front panel.

If low cardiac output causes insufficient arterial perfusion in your patient's earlobe—preventing an accurate determination of oxygen saturation with an ear oximeter—you can use a *pulse oximeter*. This instrument measures the wavelengths of light transmitted through a *pulsating* arterial vascular bed, such as in a fingertip. As the pulsating bed expands and relaxes, the light path length changes, producing a waveform. Because the waveform's produced solely from arterial blood, the pulse oximeter calculates the exact, beat-by-beat arterial oxygen saturation without interference from surrounding venous blood, skin, connective tissue, or bone. LED light emitters and a photodiode light receptor are mounted in a receptacle that you slip over your patient's fingertip (no heater is required). The receptacle is connected to a microprocessor that calculates and displays the saturation values.

You can't use the fingertip receptacle on a patient who has any condition that significantly reduces peripheral vascular pulsations (such as hypothermia or hypotension) or who's taking vasoactive drugs. Instead, you'll use a nasal probe that fits around your patient's septal anterior ethmoid artery, where vascular pulsations are less easily disrupted.

Areas of Auscultation

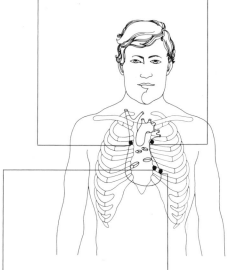

Aortic area (second right intercostal space, close to the sternum)

Pulmonic area (second left intercostal space, close to the sternum)

Tricuspid area (fifth left intercostal space, lower left sternal border)

Mitral (apical) area (fifth left intercostal space, medial to the midclavicular line)

Chest Auscultation: Listening for Heart Sounds

S₁

Timing
Beginning of systole
Physiology
Mitral and tricuspid valves close almost simultaneously, producing a single sound; S₁ corresponds to the carotid pulse.
Indication
● Normal
Where to auscultate
Apex

ACCENTUATED S₁

Timing
Beginning of systole
Physiology
Mitral valve is still open wide at the beginning of systole, so the valve slams shut from an open position.
Indication
● During rapid heart rate
● Mitral stenosis
● After mitral valve disease, such as mitral prolapse
Where to auscultate
Apex

DIMINISHED S₁

Timing
Beginning of systole
Physiology
Mitral valve floats to an almost-closed position before ventricular contraction shuts it, so it closes less forcefully.
Indication
● First-degree heart block
● Mitral regurgitation
● Severe mitral stenosis with calcified immobile valve
Where to auscultate
Apex

SPLIT S₁

Timing
Beginning of systole
Physiology
Mitral valve closes slightly before the tricuspid valve.
Indication
● Normal in most cases
● Right bundle-branch heart block (wide splitting of S₁)
● Pulmonary hypertension
Where to auscultate
Beginning at mitral area and moving toward tricuspid area
Continued

Chest Auscultation: Listening for Heart Sounds
Continued

S₂

Timing
End of systole
Physiology
Pulmonic and aortic valves close almost simultaneously.
Indication
• Normal
Where to auscultate
Aortic and pulmonic areas (base); heard best at aortic area

PHYSIOLOGIC SPLIT S₂
(Split on inspiration but not on expiration)

Timing
End of systole
Physiology
During inspiration, the pulmonic valve closes later than the aortic valve. (Pulmonic valve closure is normally delayed during inspiration, which causes decreased thoracic pressure and allows more blood into the right side of the heart, delaying pulmonic valve closure.)

Indication
• Normal; a physiologic S₂ split corresponds to the respiratory cycle
Where to auscultate
Aortic and pulmonic areas; heard best at pulmonic area on inspiration

---

PERSISTENT WIDE SPLIT S₂ (split on both inspiration and expiration, but more widely split on inspiration)

Timing
End of systole
Physiology
Pulmonic valve closes late or (less commonly) the aortic valve closes early.
Indication
Late pulmonic valve closure:
• Complete right bundle-branch heart block, which delays right ventricular contraction. As a result, the pulmonic valve closes later
• Pulmonary stenosis, which prolongs right ventricular ejection
Where to auscultate
Pulmonic area

Continued

Chest Auscultation: Listening for Heart Sounds
Continued

FIXED SPLIT S$_2$ (equally split on inspiration and expiration)

Timing
End of systole

Physiology
Pulmonic valve consistently closes later than aortic valve. Right side of heart is already ejecting a larger volume, so filling cannot be increased during inspiration. The sound remains fixed.

Indication
• Severe right ventricular failure, which prolongs right ventricular systole
• Atrial septal defect, which causes blood return to the right ventricle from lungs, prolonging the ejection

Where to auscultate
Pulmonic area

PARADOXICAL (REVERSED) S$_2$ SPLIT (widely split on expiration)

Timing
End of systole

Physiology
On expiration, aortic valve closes after the pulmonic valve from delayed or prolonged left ventricular systole. On inspiration, the normal delay of the pulmonic valve closure causes the two sounds to merge.

Indication
• Left bundle-branch heart block (most common cause)
• Aortic stenosis
• Patent ductus arteriosus
• Severe hypertension
• Left ventricular failure, disease, or ischemia

Where to auscultate
Aortic area

S$_3$ (ventricular gallop)

Timing
Early diastole

Physiology
Ventricles fill early and rapidly, causing vibrations of the ventricular walls.

Indication
• Early congestive heart failure
• Ventricular aneurysm
• Common in children and young adults

Continued

Chest Auscultation: Listening for Heart Sounds
Continued

S$_3$ (ventricular gallop)
Continued

Where to auscultate
Mitral area and right ventricular area, using stethoscope bell, with patient on his left side

S$_4$ (atrial gallop)

Timing
Late diastole
Physiology
Atrium makes an extra effort to fill against increased resistance.
Indication
• Hypertensive cardiovascular disease
• Chronic coronary artery disease
• Aortic stenosis
• Hypertrophic cardiomyopathy
• Pulmonary artery hypertension
Where to auscultate
Apex

CARDIOVASCULAR CARE

Nursing Tip

Remember these important points when performing an initial assessment on a critically ill patient:
1. Collect assessment information from the patient that includes his history and profile, perform a thorough physical examination, and obtain baseline laboratory data.
2. Consider your patient's vital signs a valuable indicator of trends or possible future changes, as well as an index of his present condition.
3. Keep your assessment accurate and fast by following a systematic approach.
4. Be aware that a change in pulse pressure may signal increasing intracranial pressure or shock.

What Your Inspection and Palpation Findings Mean

CARDIOVASCULAR CARE

INSPECTION AND PALPATION AREA/ POSSIBLE OBSERVATIONS	POSSIBLE ABNORMALITIES
Sternoclavicular	
• Abnormally strong pulsation	• Aortic aneurysm
Aortic	
• Abnormally abrupt pulsation	• Rheumatic heart disease • Systemic hypertension
• Thrill	• Aortic stenosis
Pulmonary	
• Abnormally abrupt pulsation	• Essential pulmonary hypertension
• Thrill	• Pulmonic stenosis
• Abnormally strong or forceful pulsation	• Emphysema, mitral stenosis • Extensive pneumonia • Pulmonary embolism
Right ventricular	
• Thrill	• Ventricular septal defect
• Heave and lift with each heartbeat	• Right ventricular hypertrophy • Pulmonic stenosis • Systemic hypertension • Emphysema, mitral stenosis • Extensive pneumonia

Continued

What Your Inspection and Palpation Findings Mean
Continued

INSPECTION AND PALPATION AREA/ POSSIBLE OBSERVATIONS	POSSIBLE ABNORMALITIES
Left ventricular	
• Thrill	• Mitral stenosis
• Gallop	• Ischemia • Injury • Myocardial infarction
• Impulse far to the left or low	• Aortic regurgitation • Aortic stenosis • Left ventricular hypertrophy • Systemic hypertension
• Impulse covering a large area	• Aortic regurgitation • Aortic stenosis • Left ventricular hypertrophy • Systemic hypertension
• Impulse long in duration and/or abnormally strong	• Aortic regurgitation • Aortic stenosis • Left ventricular hypertrophy • Systemic hypertension
Epigastric	
• Abnormally strong pulsation	• Aortic aneurysm

Assessing Chest Pain

CONDITION/LOCATION AND RADIATION	CHARACTER
Myocardial ischemia (angina pectoris) • Substernal or retrosternal pain spreading across chest • May radiate to inside of either or both arms, the neck, or jaw	• Squeezing, heavy pressure, aching, or burning discomfort
Myocardial infarction • Substernal or over precordium • May radiate throughout chest and arms to jaw	• Crushing, viselike, steady pain
Pericardial chest pain • Substernal or left of sternum • May radiate to neck, arms, back, or epigastrium	Sharp, intermittent pain (accentuated by swallowing, coughing, deep inspiration, or lying supine)
Pulmonary embolism • Inferior portion of the pleura • May radiate to costal margins or upper abdomen	• Stabbing, knifelike pain (accentuated by respirations)

CARDIOVASCULAR CARE

ONSET AND DURATION	PRECIPITATING EVENTS	ASSOCIATED FINDINGS
• Sudden onset • Usually subsides within 5 minutes	• Mental or physical exertion; intense emotion • Heavy food intake; especially in extreme temperatures or high humidity	• Feeling of uneasiness or impending doom
• Sudden onset • More severe and prolonged than anginal pain	• Occurs spontaneously, with exertion, stress, or at rest	• Dyspnea • Profuse perspiration • Nausea and vomiting • Dizziness, weakness • Feeling of uneasiness or impending doom
• Severe, sudden onset • Usually relieved by bending forward • May occur intermittently over several days	• Upper respiratory tract infection • Myocardial infarction • Rheumatic fever • Pericarditis	• Distended neck veins • Tachycardia • Paradoxical pulse possible with constrictive pericarditis • Pericardial friction rub
• Sudden onset • May last a few days	• Anxiety (associated with coughing)	• Dyspnea; tachypnea • Tachycardia • Cough with hemoptysis

Continued

Assessing Chest Pain
Continued

CONDITION/LOCATION AND RADIATION	CHARACTER
Spontaneous pneumothorax • Lateral thorax • Does not radiate	• Tearing, pleuritic pain
Infectious or inflammatory processes (pleurisy) • Pleural • May be widespread or only over affected area	• Moderate, sharp, raw, burning pain
Aortic (dissecting aortic aneurysm) • Anterior chest • May radiate to thoracic portion of back	• Excruciating, knifelike pain
Esophageal pain • Substernal • May radiate around chest to shoulders	• Burning, knotlike pain (simulating angina)
Chest wall pain • Costochondral or sternocostal junctions • Does not radiate	• Aching pain or soreness

ONSET AND DURATION	PRECIPITATING EVENTS	ASSOCIATED FINDINGS
• Sudden onset • Relieved by aspiration of air	• Trauma • Ruptured emphysematous bleb • Anxiety	• Dyspnea; tachypnea • Mediastinal shift • Decreased or absent breath sounds
• Occurs on inspiration • Relief usually occurs several days after treatment	• Underlying disease of lung, such as pneumonia	• Fever • Cough with sputum production
• Sudden onset • Unrelieved by medication or comfort measures • May last for hours	• Hypertension	• Lower blood pressure in one arm than in other • May have pulsus paradoxus • Hypotension and shock
• Sudden onset • Relieved by diet or position change, antacids, or belching • Usually brief duration	• May occur spontaneously • Eating	• Regurgitation
• Often begins as dull ache, worsening over a few days • Usually long lasting	• Chest wall movement	• Symptoms and physical findings vary with specific musculoskeletal disorder

EKG Leads: A Closer Look

You can think of an EKG's 12 leads as independent television cameras, each focused on the same subject but viewing it from a different angle. The chart below lists each lead with corresponding direction of electrical potential and view of the heart. The normal EKG waveforms for each of the 12 leads are shown below right.

STANDARD LIMB LEADS
(Bipolar)

Lead I

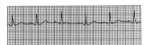

Direction of electrical potential
Between left arm (positive pole) and right arm (negative pole)
View of heart
Lateral wall

Lead II

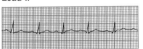

Direction of electrical potential
Between left leg (positive pole) and right arm (negative pole)
View of heart
Inferior wall

Lead III

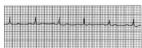

Direction of electrical potential
Between left leg (positive pole) and left arm (negative pole)
View of heart
Inferior wall

AUGMENTED LIMB LEADS
(Unipolar)

Lead aVR

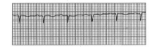

Direction of electrical potential
Right arm to heart
View of heart
Provides no specific view

Lead aVL

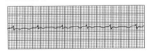

Direction of electrical potential
Left arm to heart
View of heart
Lateral wall

Continued

EKG Leads: A Closer Look
Continued

AUGMENTED LIMB LEADS
Continued

Lead aVF

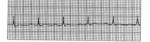

Direction of electrical potential
Left foot to heart
View of heart
Inferior wall

PRECORDIAL, OR CHEST,
LEADS (Unipolar)

Lead V₁

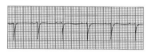

Direction of electrical potential
Fourth intercostal space, right
sternal border, to heart
View of heart
Anteroseptal wall

Lead V₂

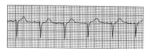

Direction of electrical potential
Fourth intercostal space, left ster-
nal border, to heart
View of heart
Anteroseptal wall

Lead V₃

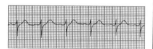

Direction of electrical potential
Midway between V_2 and V_4 to
heart
View of heart
Anterior wall

Lead V₄

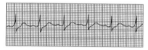

Direction of electrical potential
Fifth intercostal space, midclavic-
ular line, to heart
View of heart
Anterior wall

Continued

EKG Leads: A Closer Look
Continued

PRECORDIAL, OR CHEST,
LEADS
Continued

Lead V₅

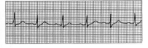

Direction of electrical potential
Fifth intercostal space, anterior
axillary line, to heart
View of heart
Lateral wall

Lead V₆

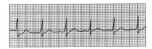

Direction of electrical potential
Fifth intercostal space, midaxillary
line, to heart
View of heart
Lateral wall

Making Waves

The waves of an EKG correlate
with the electrical stimulation that
precedes the mechanical contraction and relaxation of the heart.
These waves have arbitrarily
been labeled the P, QRS, and T
waves.

The P wave reflects depolarization of the atria and therefore is a
good indication of SA node function. The QRS complex reflects
the depolarization of the ventricles. The T wave reflects the re-
polarization of the ventricles. (The
T wave corresponding to the re-

polarization of the atria isn't visible because the QRS deflection
obscures it.) The mass of the
ventricles is much greater than
that of the atria, so the QRS and
T waves are much larger than the
P wave.

Occasionally, another wave,
called a U wave, will appear after
the T wave. The U wave may reflect electrolyte disturbances or
drug influence. However, U waves
may appear for *no* reason in
some people.

Standard 12-Lead EKG

Normally, five electrodes (four limb, one chest) record the heart's electrical potential from 12 different views (leads). One electrode serves as a ground. Standard bipolar limb leads (I, II, III) detect variations in electrical potential at two points (the negative pole and the positive pole) and record the difference. The unipolar augmented limb leads (aVR, aVL, and aVF) measure electrical potential between one augmented limb lead and the electrical midpoint of the remaining two leads. Six unipolar chest leads (V_1 through V_6) view electrical potential from a horizontal plane that helps locate pathology in the lateral and posterior walls of the heart.

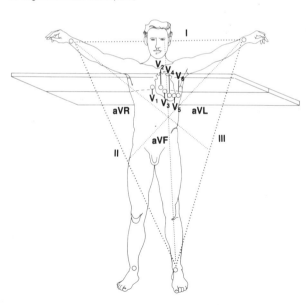

Cardiac Conduction: Following the Route

The numbers on the heart below trace the cardiac conduction route. The key below tells you which part of the heart's anatomy corresponds with each number.

1. Sinus node (SA node)
2. Intraatrial tracts
3. Atrial muscle fibers
4. Atrioventricular node (AV node)
5. Bundle of His
6. Right bundle branch
7. Superior and inferior divisions of left bundle branch
8. Purkinje's fibers
9. Ventricular muscle

As you can see, the impulse arrives first at the sinoatrial node, works its way through the heart chambers, and eventually reaches the ventricular muscle.

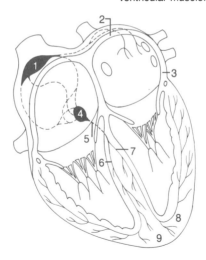

CARDIOVASCULAR CARE

Cardiac Monitoring Facts

Like other forms of electro-cardiography, cardiac monitoring uses electrodes applied to the patient's chest to pick up patterns of cardiac impulses for display and analysis on a monitor screen. The monitor displays the patient's heart rate and rhythm, sounds an alarm if the heart rate rises above or falls below the allowable per-minute setting, and provides printouts of cardiac rhythms. Cardiac monitoring allows continuous observation of the heart's electrical activity in patients with a symptomatic dysrhythmia or any cardiac pathology that might lead to life-threatening dysrhythmias. It's also used to evaluate effects of therapy.

Two types: Hardwire and telemetry monitoring
Hardwire monitoring permits continuous observation of a patient directly connected to the monitor console. In contrast, telemetry monitoring permits continuous monitoring of an ambulatory patient who isn't connected to a monitor. In telemetry monitoring, cardiac impulses travel from a small transmitter worn by the patient to antenna wires in the ceiling that relay patterns to the monitor screen. Telemetry monitoring permits greater patient mobility than hardwire monitoring, and avoids electrical hazards by isolating the monitor system from leakage and accidental shock. But telemetry monitoring is limited; its relay wires pick up the heartbeat only within 50' to 2,000' (15 to 610 m) of the central console, depending on the equipment and the unit's floor plan.

Continued

CARDIOVASCULAR CARE

Special Consideration

Avoid removing the paper backing of the electrodes until just before application *to prevent them from drying out.* Position electrodes on the patient's chest *so they won't interfere with application of defibrillator paddles if emergency defibrillation is required.*

Make sure all electrical equipment and outlets are grounded properly *to avoid electrical shock and artifacts.*

Cardiac Monitoring Facts
Continued

CARDIOVASCULAR CARE

Three-electrode monitor

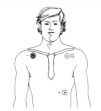

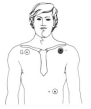

Lead II
Positive (+): left side of chest, lowest palpable rib, midclavicular line
Negative (−): right shoulder, below clavicular hollow
Ground (G): left shoulder, below clavicular hollow

MCL₆
Positive (+): left side of chest, lowest palpable rib, midclavicular line
Negative (−): left shoulder, below clavicular hollow
Ground (G): right shoulder, below clavicular hollow

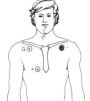

MCL₁
Positive (+): right sternal border, lowest palpable rib
Negative (−): left shoulder, below clavicular hollow
Ground (G): right shoulder, below clavicular hollow

Caring for the Patient Being Monitored

Explain the monitoring procedure to him step by step, so he knows what to expect. Tell him why he's being monitored and how it helps. Investigate what he knows about monitoring, then clear up any misconceptions. For example, is he afraid the alarm will go off when he moves? Does he think he'll get a shock from the electrodes? Anticipate such concerns and try to relieve his anxieties. Sound the alarm so he knows what to expect. Tell him that false alarms are likely. Finally, make sure the monitor doesn't face the patient.

During monitoring, don't place more importance on the monitor than on your patient. *When you enter his room, greet him first and attend to his needs before you go to the monitor.* Don't discuss his condition with others at his bedside unless you include him in the discussions, too. If the monitor sounds an alarm, fight your natural inclination to look toward the monitor. Even if you suspect that the monitor's malfunctioning—and the alarm's not an indication that the patient's condition is deteriorating—don't take any chances. First, determine without question that your patient doesn't need attention. Then, look at the equipment.

CARDIOVASCULAR CARE

Troubleshooting Cardiac Monitors

SKIN EXCORIATION UNDER ELECTRODE

Problem/possible causes
• Patient allergic to the electrode adhesive
• Electrode left on skin too long
Solution
• Remove electrodes and apply hypoallergenic electrodes and hy-

poallergenic tape.
• Remove electrode, clean site, and reapply electrode at new site. *Note:* Do this every 2 or 3 days to avoid the problem.

BROKEN LEAD WIRES OR A BROKEN CABLE

Problem/possible causes
• Stress loops not used on lead wires

Continued

Troubleshooting Cardiac Monitors
Continued

BROKEN LEAD WIRES OR A
BROKEN CABLE
Continued

• Cables and lead wires cleaned
with alcohol or acetone, causing
brittleness
Solution
• Replace lead wires and retape
them, using stress loops.
• Clean wires with soapy water,
not alcohol or acetone. *Important:*
Do not wet cable ends.

WANDERING BASELINE

Problem/possible causes
• Patient restless
• Chest wall movement during
respiration
• Improper application of elec-
trodes
• Use of nonpolarized electrodes
Solution
• Encourage patient to relax.
• Tighten electrode connections.
• Check electrodes and reapply
them, if necessary. Place elec-
trodes on fleshy, not bony, areas.
• Polarize electrodes.

STRAIGHT LINE ON MONITOR
(NOT CAUSED BY ASYSTOLE)

Problem/possible causes
• Improper connection of lead
wire to either electrode or cable

Solution
• Check cable and electrode connections and adjust them, if necessary.

FUZZY BASELINE (60- OR 50-
CYCLE INTERFERENCE)

Problem/possible causes
• Electrical interference from
other equipment in the room
• Improper grounding of patient's
bed
Solution
• Make sure all electrical equipment is attached to the patient's
common ground. Check three-
pronged plugs to make sure none
of the prongs is loose.
• Make sure the bed ground is attached to the room's common
ground.

ARTIFACT (WAVEFORM INTER-
FERENCE)

Problem/possible causes
• Patient experiencing seizures,
chills, or anxiety
• Patient restless
• Dirty or corroded connections
• Improper application of elec-
trodes
• Electrical short circuit in lead
wires or cable
• Electrical interference from
other equipment in the room
Continued

Troubleshooting Cardiac Monitors
Continued

ARTIFACT (WAVEFORM INTER-
FERENCE)
Continued

• Static electricity interference,
from decrease in room humidity
Solution
• Notify doctor if the patient's
having seizures, and treat patient,
as ordered. Keep patient warm
and reassured. Spend time with
him, and discuss his fears.
• Encourage patient to relax.
• Replace dirty or corroded wires.
• Check electrodes and reapply
them, if necessary. Take care to
clean the patient's skin thoroughly,
because skin oils and dead skin
cells interfere with conduction.
• Check electrode jelly. If the jelly's dry, apply new electrodes.
• Replace broken equipment. Use
stress loops when applying lead
wires.
• Make sure all electrical equipment is attached to a common
ground. Check three-pronged
plugs to make sure none of the
prongs are loose.
• Regulate room humidity to 40%,
if possible.

DOUBLE-TRIGGERING (P WAVE
AND QRS COMPLEX, OR QRS
COMPLEX AND T WAVE, ARE
OF EQUAL HEIGHT)

Problem/possible causes
• GAIN setting too high, particu-
larly with MCL_1 setting
Solution
• Reset GAIN. If possible, monitor
patient on MCL_6 or another lead.

ALARM SOUNDS, BUT YOU
SEE NO EVIDENCE OF DYS-
RHYTHMIA

Problem/possible causes
• Improper application of elec-
trodes
• QRS complex too small
• HIGH alarm set too low, or LOW
alarm set too high
• Artifact (waveform interference)
• Wire or cable failure
• Voltage too high or too low
Solution
• Reapply electrodes.
• Reset GAIN so that the height of
the complex is greater than 1 mil-
livolt.
• Try monitoring patient on an-
other lead.
• Set alarm limits according to
patient's heart rate.
• Check electrodes and reapply
them, if necessary.
• Replace faulty wire or cable.
• Adjust GAIN on bedside monitor.

Cardiac Dysrhythmias

NORMAL SINUS RHYTHM (N.S.R.) IN ADULTS

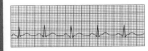

Description
• Ventricular and atrial rates of 60 to 100 beats per minute (BPM)
• QRS complexes and P waves regular and uniform
• Constant PR interval of 0.12 to 0.2 seconds
• QRS duration < 0.12 seconds
• Identical atrial and ventricular rates

SINUS ARRHYTHMIA

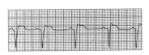

Causes
• Usually a normal variation of NSR; associated with sinus bradycardia
Description
• Slight irregularity of heart-beat, usually corresponding to respiratory cycle
• PR interval increases with inspiration and decreases with expiration
Treatment
• None

SINUS TACHYCARDIA

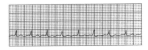

Causes
• Normal physiologic response to fever, exercise, anxiety, pain, dehydration; may also accompany shock, left ventricular failure, cardiac tamponade, anemia, hyperthyroidism, hypovolemia, pulmonary embolus
• May result from treatment with vagolytic and sympathetic stimulating drugs
Description
• Rate > 100 BPM; rarely, > 160 BPM
• Every QRS wave follows a P wave
Treatment
• Correct underlying cause

Continued

CARDIOVASCULAR CARE

Cardiac Dysrhythmias
Continued

SINUS BRADYCARDIA

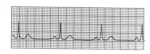

Causes
• Increased intracranial pressure; increased vagal tone due to bowel straining, vomiting, intubation, mechanical ventilation; sick sinus syndrome or hypothyroidism
• Treatment with beta-blockers and sympatholytic drugs
• May be normal in athletes

Description
• Rate: 60 BPM
• A QRS complex follows each P wave

Treatment
• For signs of low cardiac output, dizziness, weakness, altered level of consciousness, or low blood pressure, at least 0.4 mg atropine every 5 minutes
• Temporary ventricular pacemaker or isoproterenol, if atropine fails

SINOATRIAL ARREST, OR BLOCK (SINUS ARREST)

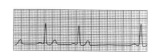

Causes
• Vagal stimulation, digitalis or quinidine toxicity
• Often a sign of sick sinus syndrome

Description
• NSR interrupted by unexpectedly prolonged P-P interval, often terminated by a junctional escape beat or return to NSR
• QRS complexes uniform but irregular

Treatment
• A pacemaker for repeated episodes

CARDIOVASCULAR CARE

Continued

Cardiac Dysrhythmias
Continued

CARDIOVASCULAR CARE

WANDERING ATRIAL PACEMAKER

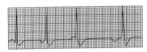

Causes
● Seen in rheumatic pancarditis as a result of inflammation involving the SA node, digitalis toxicity, sick sinus syndrome

Description
● Rate varies
● QRS complexes uniform in shape but irregular in rhythm
● P waves irregular with changing configuration, indicating they're not all from sinus node or single atrial focus
● P-R interval varies from short to normal

Treatment
● If patient is taking digitalis, discontinue
● No other treatment

PREMATURE ATRIAL CONTRACTION (P.A.C.)

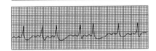

Causes
● Congestive heart failure, ischemic heart disease, acute respiratory failure, or COPD
● May result from treatment with digitalis, aminophylline, or adrenergic drugs; or from anxiety, excessive caffeine ingestion
● Occasional PAC may be normal

Description
● Premature, occasionally abnormal-looking P waves
● QRS complexes follow, except in very early or blocked PACs
● P wave often buried in the preceding T wave or can often be identified in the preceding T wave

Treatment
● If more than six times per minute or frequency is increasing, give digitalis, quinidine, or propranolol
● Eliminate known causes, such as caffeine or drugs

Continued

Cardiac Dysrhythmias
Continued

PAROXYSMAL ATRIAL
TACHYCARDIA (P.A.T.), OR
PAROXYSMAL SUPRAVEN-
TRICULAR TACHYCARDIA

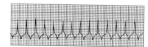

Causes
● Intrinsic abnormality of AV
conduction system
● Congenital accessory atrial
conduction pathway
● Physical or psychological
stress, hypoxia, hypokalemia,
caffeine, marijuana, stimu-
lants, digitalis toxicity
Description
● Heart rate > 140 BPM;
rarely exceeds 250 BPM
● P waves regular but aberrant; difficult to differentiate
from preceding T wave
● Onset and termination of
dysrhythmia occur suddenly
● May cause palpitations and
light-headedness
Treatment
● Vagal maneuvers, sympa-
thetic blockers, or calcium
blockers to alter AV node
conduction

● Elective cardioversion, if patient is symptomatic and unre-
sponsive to drugs

ATRIAL FLUTTER

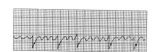

Causes
● Heart failure, valvular heart
disease, pulmonary embolism,
digitalis toxicity, postoperative
revascularization
Description
● Ventricular rate depends on
degree of AV block (usually 60
to 100 BPM)
● Atrial rate 240 to 400 BPM
and regular
● QRS complexes uniform in
shape, but often irregular in rate
● P waves may have saw-
tooth configuration
Treatment
● Digitalis (unless dysrhythmia is due to digitalis toxicity), propranolol, or quinidine
● May require synchronized
cardioversion, atrial pacemaker, or vagal stimulation

Continued

Cardiac Dysrhythmias
Continued

ATRIAL FIBRILLATION

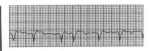

NODAL RHYTHM (A.V. JUNCTIONAL RHYTHM)

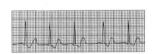

Causes
• Congestive heart failure, COPD, hyperthyroidism, sepsis, pulmonary embolus, mitral stenosis, digitalis toxicity (rarely), atrial irritation, post-coronary bypass or valve replacement surgery

Description
• Atrial rate > 400 BPM
• Ventricular rate varies
• QRS complexes uniform in shape, but at irregular intervals
• P-R interval indiscernible
• No P waves, or P waves appear as erratic, irregular baseline F waves
• Irregular QRS rate

Treatment
• Digitalis and quinidine to slow ventricular rate, and quinidine to convert rhythm to NSR; diuretics, such as furosemide, for congestive heart failure
• May require elective cardioversion for rapid rate

Causes
• Digitalis toxicity, inferior wall myocardial infarction or ischemia, hypoxia, vagal stimulation
• Acute rheumatic fever
• Valve surgery

Description
• Ventricular rate usually 40 to 60 BPM (60 to 100 BPM is accelerated junctional rhythm)
• P waves may precede, be hidden within (absent), or follow QRS; if visible, they're altered
• QRS duration is normal, except in aberrant conduction.
• Patient may be asymptomatic unless ventricular rate is very slow

Treatment
• Symptomatic
• Atropine, with slow rate
• If patient is taking digitalis, discontinue

Continued

Cardiac Dysrhythmias
Continued

PREMATURE NODAL CONTRACTIONS (P.N.C.), OR JUNCTIONAL PREMATURE BEATS

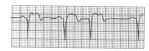

Causes
● Myocardial infarction or ischemia, digitalis toxicity, excessive caffeine ingestion
Description
● Underlying rhythm is sinus or atrial
● QRS complexes of uniform shape but irregular rate
● P waves irregular, with premature beat; may precede, be hidden within, or follow QRS
Treatment
● Correct underlying cause
● Quinidine or disopyramide, as ordered
● If patient is taking digitalis, discontinue

FIRST-DEGREE A.V. BLOCK

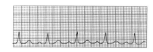

Causes
● Inferior myocardial ischemia or infarction, hypothyroidism, digitalis toxicity, potassium imbalance
Description
● P-R interval prolonged > 0.2 seconds
● QRS complex normal
Treatment
● If patient is taking digitalis, discontinue
● Correct underlying cause; otherwise, be alert for increasing block

Continued

Cardiac Dysrhythmias
Continued

SECOND-DEGREE A.V. BLOCK (MOBITZ TYPE I: WENCKEBACH)

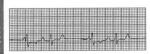

Causes
• *Mobitz Type I:* Inferior wall myocardial infarction, digitalis toxicity, vagal stimulation
Description
• *Mobitz Type I:* P-R interval becomes progressively longer with each cycle until QRS disappears (dropped beat). After a dropped beat, P-R interval is shorter. Ventricular rate is irregular; atrial rhythm, regular
Treatment
• *Mobitz Type I:* atropine if patient is symptomatic
• Discontinue digitalis

SECOND-DEGREE A.V. BLOCK (MOBITZ TYPE II)

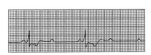

Causes
• *Mobitz Type II:* Degenerative disease of conduction system, ischemia of AV node in anterior myocardial infarction, digitalis toxicity, anteroseptal infarction
Description
• *Mobitz Type II:* P-R interval is constant, with QRS complex dropped at regular intervals
• Ventricular rhythm may be irregular, with varying degree of block
• Atrial rate regular
Treatment
• *Mobitz Type II:* temporary pacemaker, sometimes followed by permanent pacemaker
• Atropine, for slow rate
• If patient is taking digitalis, discontinue

Continued

Cardiac Dysrhythmias
Continued

THIRD-DEGREE A.V. BLOCK (COMPLETE HEART BLOCK)

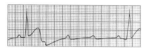

Causes
● Ischemic heart disease or infarction; postsurgical complications of mitral valve replacement; digitalis toxicity; hypoxia sometimes causing syncope due to decreased cerebral blood flow, as in Stokes-Adams syndrome
Description
● Atrial rate regular; ventricular rate slow and regular
● No relationship between P waves and QRS complexes
● No constant P-R interval
● QRS interval normal (nodal pacemaker); wide and bizarre (ventricular pacemaker)
Treatment
● Usually requires temporary pacemaker, followed by permanent pacemaker
● Epinephrine or isoproterenol

NODAL TACHYCARDIA (JUNCTIONAL TACHYCARDIA)

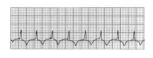

Causes
● Digitalis toxicity, myocarditis, cardiomyopathy, myocardial ischemia or infarct
Description
● Onset of rhythm often sudden, occurring in bursts
● Ventricular rate > 100 BPM
● Other characteristics same as junctional rhythm
Treatment
● Vagal stimulation
● Propranolol, quinidine, digitalis (if cause is not digitalis toxicity)
● Elective cardioversion

PREMATURE VENTRICULAR CONTRACTION (P.V.C.)

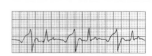

Continued

Cardiac Dysrhythmias
Continued

PREMATURE VENTRICU-
LAR CONTRACTION (P.V.C.)
Continued

Causes
● Heart failure; old or acute
myocardial infarction or contusion with trauma; myocardial irritation by ventricular catheter;
hypoxia; drug toxicity (digitalis,
aminophylline, tricyclic antide-
pressants, beta-adrenergics);
electrolyte imbalances (especially hypokalemia); stress
Description
● Beat occurs prematurely,
usually followed by a complete compensatory pause after PVC; irregular pulse
● QRS complex wide and dis-
torted
● Can occur singly, in pairs,
or in threes; and can alter-
nate with normal beats
● Focus can be from one or
more sites
● PVCs are most ominous
when clustered and multifo-
cal, with R wave on T pattern
Treatment
● Lidocaine I.V. bolus and
drip infusion; procainamide
I.V. If induced by digitalis toxicity, stop this drug; if induced by

hypokalemia, give potassium
chloride I.V.

VENTRICULAR TACHYCAR-
DIA (V.T.)

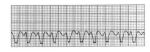

Causes
● Myocardial ischemia, infarction, or aneurysm; ventricular
catheters; digitalis or quinidine toxicity; hypokalemia;
hypercalcemia; anxiety
Description
● Ventricular rate 140 to 220
BPM; may be regular
● QRS complexes are wide,
bizarre, and independent of P
waves
● No visible P waves
● Can produce chest pain,
dyspnea, shock, coma, and
death
Treatment
● CPR (if cardiac arrest occurs), followed by lidocaine
I.V. (bolus and drip infusion);
synchronized cardioversion
● For recurrent episodes, use
bretylium tosylate

Continued

Cardiac Dysrhythmias
Continued

VENTRICULAR FIBRILLATION

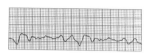

Causes
• Myocardial ischemia or infarction, untreated ventricular tachycardia, electrolyte imbalances (hypokalemia and alkalosis, hyperkalemia and hypercalcemia), digitalis or quinidine toxicity, electric shock, hypothermia

Description
• Ventricular rhythm rapid and chaotic
• QRS complexes are wide and irregular; no visible P waves
• Loss of consciousness with no peripheral pulses, blood pressure, or respirations; possible seizures; and sudden death

Treatment
• CPR
• Asynchronized countershock (400 watts/second). If rhythm doesn't return, shock again
• Drugs, such as lidocaine or bretylium tosylate I.V. (for recurrent episodes)

VENTRICULAR STANDSTILL (ASYSTOLE)

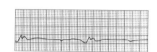

Causes
• Acute respiratory failure, myocardial ischemia or infarction, ruptured ventricular aneurysm, aortic valve disease, or hyperkalemia

Description
• Primary ventricular standstill—regular P waves, no QRS complexes
• Secondary ventricular standstill—QRS complexes wide and slurred, occurring at irregular intervals; agonal heart rhythm
• Loss of consciousness with no peripheral pulses, blood pressure, or respirations

Treatment
• CPR
• Endotracheal intubation; pacemaker should be available
• Epinephrine, calcium gluconate, and sodium bicarbonate
• Cardiac monitoring

Assisting with Elective Cardioversion

Like defibrillation, elective cardioversion attempts to restore the sinoatrial node to its function as the heart's natural pacemaker.

To prepare for cardioversion, assemble all the equipment for defibrillation, including an EKG monitor, I.V. infusion equipment, a cardioverter with synchronizer, an emergency drug cart, and suction equipment.

Next make sure the patient or a responsible family member understands cardioversion and signs a consent form. Instruct the patient to abstain from food and fluids for at least 7 or 8 hours, and withhold digitalis for 24 to 36 hours. If you suspect digitalis toxicity, the doctor will probably order the patient's digitalis level taken. Cardioversion usually is delayed until the digitalis level is normal. In many institutions a potassium blood level is obtained and documented prior to this procedure.

Start a peripheral I.V. to administer a sedative or emergency drugs, as ordered. Attach the patient to the EKG monitor and run a 12-lead tracing to detect dysrhythmias. Leave the limb electrodes in place for later recordings. Place chest electrodes in position to obtain the tallest R wave; in most patients this chest lead would be modified lead II or

MCL. Make sure the electrodes don't interfere with cardioverter paddle placement. Attach the cardioverter to the monitor and turn on the synchronizer switch or button. Make sure the synchronizer artifact falls on the R wave; *if the cardioverter doesn't recognize the R wave, it won't discharge.* To increase the R wave, increase sensitivity, but make sure not to increase the T wave to the height where the cardioverter recognizes it; or select another lead that shows a larger R wave.

Place the patient in a supine position, and avoid raising the head more than 30°. Have an emergency crash cart ready in case symptomatic bradycardia or ventricular dysrhythmias occur. If the patient has loosely fitting dentures, remove them to prevent airway obstruction after sedation. However, if they fit properly, leave them in place to make airway management easier.

Bare the male patient's chest, but cover the female patient's breasts with a towel until paddle electrodes are in position. Administer a sedative, as ordered.

Set the energy level on the cardioverter as ordered (usually 25 or 50 joules). Lubricate the A/P paddle electrodes as for defibrillation. The doctor should now be

Continued

Assisting with Elective Cardioversion
Continued

present to check the patient's sedation level and to perform cardioversion. Make sure the patient is adequately ventilated, and record baseline vital signs prior to cardioversion, *because the sedative may cause apnea or hypotension.*

Make sure the cardioverter is still synchronized with the R wave. Push the charge button to raise the machine to the prescribed energy level. (Most machines have a needle indicator that shows energy level.) Turn on the strip chart recorder *to document the cardioversion.* Also document a strip that validates synchronization of electric impulse with the R wave prior to cardioversion.

If you're performing the procedure, apply A/P paddles. Put the flat paddle under the patient's body, behind the heart and slightly below the left scapula. Place the other paddle over the left precordium, directly over the heart. Apply 20 to 25 pounds of pressure to the electrodes *to ensure good skin contact and to prevent burns.* Announce "Ready; stand back," making sure everyone present is away from the bed *to prevent inadvertent grounding and shocks.*

Depress the discharge button on the anterior paddle electrode, and hold that position until the energy is delivered. (You may have to hold the button a second or more.) Remove the paddle electrodes immediately after the shock. Make sure a normal sinus rhythm is present; if it is not, repeat the procedure at a higher energy level, as ordered.

Take a 12-lead EKG and compare it to the preconversion (baseline) EKG. Take the patient's vital signs immediately after cardioversion and every 15 minutes for at least 1 hour or until stable, and observe his level of consciousness. Make sure his respiratory rate and excursive movements are adequate until he is alert. Observe the cardiac monitor pattern until rhythm stabilizes. Watch for complications of cardioversion: ventricular fibrillation, asystole, rhythm disturbances, skin burns, pulmonary edema or embolus, respiratory depression or arrest, hypotension, and ST segment changes.

When the patient is alert and his condition permits, tell him he may begin to eat and move about.

Understanding Cardiac Catheterization

Simply stated, cardiac catheterization is the passing of a catheter into the right or the left side of the heart. Catheterization can determine blood pressure and blood flow in the chambers of the heart, permit collection of blood samples, or record films of the heart's ventricles (contrast ventriculography) or arteries (coronary arteriography or angiography).

In left heart catheterization, a catheter is inserted into an artery in the antecubital fossa or into the femoral artery through a puncture or cutdown procedure and, guided by fluoroscopy, the catheter is advanced retrograde through the aorta into the coronary artery orifices and/or left ventricle. Then, injection of a contrast medium into the ventricle permits radiographic visualization of the ventricle and the coronary arteries, and filming (cineangiography) of heart activity. Left heart catheterization assesses the patency of the coronary arteries, mitral and aortic valve function, and left ventricular function; it aids diagnosis of left ventricular enlargement, aortic stenosis, and regurgitation, aortic root enlargement, mitral regurgitation, aneurysm and intracardiac shunt.

In right heart catheterization, the catheter is inserted into an antecubital vein or into the femoral vein and advanced through the inferior vena cava or right atrium into the right side of the heart, and into the pulmonary artery. Right heart catheterization assesses tricuspid and pulmonary valve function and pulmonary artery pressures.

Catheterization permits blood pressure measurement in the heart chambers to determine valve competency and cardiac wall contractility, and to detect intracardiac shunts. If thermodilution catheters are used, it allows calculation of cardiac output.

Preparing Your Patient for Cardiac Catheterization

The doctor will do cardiac catheterization in a special lab, or in the ICU (if your hospital has a portable flouroscopy unit). Your responsibility is to care for the patient before and after the procedure.

Prepare the patient as soon as he's scheduled for the procedure.

• Expect to temporarily discontinue cardioactive medication.

• If the patient's scheduled for *right-sided* heart catheterization, discontinue anticoagulant therapy, according to the doctor's orders. Doing so reduces the risk of complications from venous bleeding.

• If the patient's scheduled for *left-sided* heart catheterization, continue or begin anticoagulant therapy, according to the doctor's orders. By doing this, you reduce the risk of clotting at the catheter tip, a common problem with arterial catheters.

• Explain the procedure to the patient and answer his questions. Tell him he may wear his glasses and dentures during the procedure.

• Make sure the patient's signed a consent form.

• If the procedure's scheduled for early morning, don't let your patient eat or drink anything for breakfast. But, if it's scheduled for late morning, the doctor may permit a clear liquid breakfast. These precautions reduce the risk of vomiting during the procedure, especially if the patient undergoes angiography.

• If your patient's scheduled for angiography, ask him if he has any allergies, especially an allergy to fish or iodine. If so, tell the doctor at once. Since the dye used for angiography has an iodine base, such a patient may suffer anaphylaxis when the dye's injected.

• If the insertion site's at the patient's groin or another hairy area, expect to shave his skin.

• If the doctor orders, establish an I.V. line of 5% dextrose in water or normal saline solution at keep-vein-open (KVO) rate. This will allow the doctor to give antiarrhythmic medication quickly, if necessary.

CARDIOVASCULAR CARE

Guide to Cardiac Catheterization Complications

When your patient returns from the cath lab, do you know what complications to look for? Use this chart to review your skills.

As you know, cardiac catheterization imposes more risks than most other diagnostic tests. Although the possibility of complications is slight, some of the complications can be life-threatening. That's why you must watch your patient closely during the first 48 hours after the procedure.

Keep in mind that some complications are common to *both* left- and right-sided heart catheterization; others result only from catheterization of one side.

Note: An anaphylactic reaction to the contrast dye used for angiography may occur within 15 minutes of dye injection. Since this complication occurs in the cath lab, we haven't included it in this chart.

POSSIBLE COMPLICATION OF EITHER LEFT- OR RIGHT-SIDED CATHETERIZATION

MYOCARDIAL INFARCTION

Possible cause
• Emotional stress induced by procedure
• Catheter tip dislodged blood clot, which traveled to a coronary artery (left-sided catheterization only)
Signs and symptoms
• Chest pain, possibly radiating to left arm, back, and/or jaw
• Cardiac dysrhythmias
• Diaphoresis, restlessness, and/or anxiety
• Thready pulse
• Temperature rise
• Peripheral cyanosis, causing cool skin
Nursing considerations
• Call for a code team and begin CPR, if necessary.
• Notify doctor.
• Give oxygen and other drugs, as ordered.
• Monitor patient's heart rate closely.
• Document complication and treatment.

DYSRHYTHMIAS

Possible cause
• Cardiac tissue irritated by catheter
Signs and symptoms
• Irregular heartbeat
• Irregular apical pulse
• Palpitations
Nursing considerations
• Notify doctor.

Continued

Guide to Cardiac Catheterization Complications
Continued

DYSRHYTHMIAS
Continued

• Monitor patient continuously, as ordered.
• Administer antiarrhythmic drugs, if ordered.
• Document complication and treatment.

CARDIAC TAMPONADE

Possible cause
• Perforation of heart wall by catheter
Signs and symptoms
• Dysrhythmias
• Increased heart rate
• Decreased blood pressure
• Chest pain
• Diaphoresis
• Cyanosis
Nursing considerations
• Notify doctor.
• Give oxygen, if ordered.
• Prepare patient for emergency surgery, if ordered.
• Monitor patient continuously, as ordered.
• Document complication and treatment.

INFECTION (SYSTEMIC)

Possible cause
• Poor aseptic technique
• Catheter contaminated during manufacturing process, storage, or use
Signs and symptoms
• Fever
• Increased pulse rate
• Chills and tremors
• Unstable blood pressure
Nursing considerations
• Notify doctor.
• Collect urine, sputum, and blood for culture, as ordered.
• Document complication and treatment.

HYPOVOLEMIA

Possible cause
• Diuresis from angiography dye
Signs and symptoms
• Increased urine output
• Hypotension
Nursing considerations
• Replace fluids with one or two glasses of water every hour, or maintain I.V. at a rate of 150 to 200 ml/hour, as ordered.

Continued

Guide to Cardiac Catheterization Complications
Continued

HYPOVOLEMIA
Continued

- Monitor fluid intake and output closely.
- Document complication and treatment.

HEMATOMA OR BLOOD LOSS AT INSERTION SITE

Possible cause
- Bleeding at insertion site from vein or artery damage

Signs and symptoms
- Bloody dressing
- Limb swelling
- Decreased blood pressure
- Increased heart rate

Nursing considerations
- Elevate limb and apply direct manual pressure.
- When the bleeding's stopped, apply a pressure bandage.
- If bleeding continues or if vital signs are unstable, notify doctor.
- Document complication and treatment.

POSSIBLE COMPLICATION OF EITHER LEFT- OR RIGHT-SIDED CATHETERIZATION

DYE REACTION

Possible cause
- Allergy to iodine base of angiography dye

Signs and symptoms
- Fever
- Agitation
- Hives and itching
- Decreased urine output

Nursing considerations
- Notify doctor.
- Administer antihistamines, as ordered.
- Give diuretics, as ordered.
- Monitor fluid intake and output.
- Document complication and treatment.

INFECTION AT INSERTION SITE

Possible cause
- Poor aseptic technique

Signs and symptoms
- Swelling, warmth, redness, and soreness at site.
- Purulent discharge at site

Continued

Guide to Cardiac Catheterization Complications
Continued

INFECTION AT INSERTION SITE *Continued*

Nursing considerations
• Obtain drainage sample for culture.
• Clean site and apply antimicrobial ointment, if ordered. Cover site with sterile gauze.
• Record problem and treatment.

POSSIBLE COMPLICATION OF RIGHT-SIDED CATHETERIZATION

THROMBOPHLEBITIS

Possible cause
• Vein damaged during catheter insertion
Signs and symptoms
• Vein is hard, reddened, sore, cordlike, and warm to the touch
• Swelling at site
Nursing considerations
• Elevate limb and apply warm, wet compresses.
• Notify doctor.
• Administer anticoagulant or fibrinolytic drugs, if ordered.
• Record problem and treatment.

PULMONARY EMBOLISM

Possible cause
• Catheter tip dislodged blood clot or plaque, which traveled to lungs
Signs and symptoms
• Shortness of breath
• Hyperventilation
• Increased heart rate
• Chest pain
Nursing considerations
• Notify doctor.
• Place patient in high Fowler position.
• Administer oxygen, if ordered.
• Monitor vital signs.
• Document complication and treatment.

VAGAL RESPONSE

Possible cause
• Vagus nerve endings irritated in sinoatrial (SA) node, atrial muscle tissue, or atrioventricular (AV) junction
Signs and symptoms
• Hypotension
• Decreased heart rate

Continued

Guide to Cardiac Catheterization Complications
Continued

CARDIOVASCULAR CARE

VAGAL RESPONSE
Continued

- Nausea
Nursing considerations
- Notify doctor.
- Monitor heart rate closely.
- Administer atropine.
- Keep patient supine and quiet.
- Document complication and treatment.

POSSIBLE COMPLICATION OF LEFT-SIDED CATHETERIZATION

ARTERIAL EMBOLUS OR THROMBUS IN LIMB

Possible cause
- Injury to artery during catheter insertion, causing blood clot
- Catheter dislodged plaque from artery wall
Signs and symptoms
- Slow or faint pulse distal to insertion site
- Loss of warmth, sensation, and color in limb distal to insertion site
Nursing considerations
- Notify doctor. He may perform an arteriotomy and Fo-

garty catheterization to remove embolus or thrombus.
- Protect affected limb from pressure. Keep it at room temperature and maintain it in a level or slightly dependent position.
- Administer vasodilators such as papaverine hydrochloride to relieve painful vasospasm, if ordered.
- Document complication and treatment.

CEREBROVASCULAR ACCIDENT (C.V.A.)

Possible cause
- Catheter tip dislodged blood clot or plaque, which traveled to brain
Signs and symptoms
- Hemiplegia; lethargy
- Aphasia
- Confusion, or decreased consciousness level
Nursing considerations
- Notify doctor.
- Monitor vital signs closely.
- Keep suctioning equipment nearby.
- Give oxygen, as ordered.
- Document complication and treatment.

Pulmonary Artery (PA) Catheter Insertion

After you've set up the monitoring equipment, the doctor may insert the pulmonary artery (PA) catheter percutaneously into your patient's median basilic vein. Or he may choose the subclavian, internal jugular, or femoral vein instead, depending on the patient's condition. After insertion, he'll ease the catheter further into the patient's vein until it passes through the right side of the heart and enters the pulmonary artery.

Examine these illustrations. They'll show you the route the catheter travels from the right atrium to the pulmonary artery. In addition, they'll show you how the monitor's waveform changes as the catheter progresses. The doctor depends on these waveforms to tell him the catheter tip's location. As he works, he'll expect you to record the pressure in each location.

RIGHT ATRIAL (R.A.) PRESSURE

Normal range
Mean: 3 to 6 mm Hg
1. When the tip of the PA catheter reaches your patient's right atrium from the superior vena cava, the waveform on the oscilloscope screen or readout strip will look like this. When it does, the doctor will inflate the catheter's balloon, which will float the tip through the tricuspid valve and into the right ventricle.

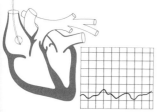

RIGHT VENTRICULAR (R.V.) PRESSURE

Normal range
Systolic: 17 to 32 mm Hg
Diastolic: 1 to 7 mm Hg
2. When the catheter tip reaches the patient's right ventricle, the waveform will look like this.

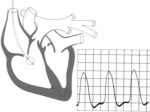

Continued

Pulmonary Artery (PA) Catheter Insertion
Continued

PULMONARY ARTERY
PRESSURE (P.A.P.)

Normal range
Systolic: 17 to 32 mm Hg
Diastolic: 4 to 13 mm Hg
Mean: 9 to 19 mm Hg
3. A waveform like this one indicates that the balloon has floated the catheter tip through the pulmonic valve into the pulmonary artery.

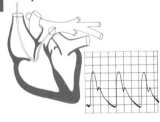

When the vessel becomes too narrow for the balloon to pass through, the balloon wedges in the vessel, occluding it. The monitor will then display a pulmonary artery wedge pressure (PAWP) waveform like this one.
Note: This pressure is sometimes called pulmonary capillary wedge pressure (PCWP), or pulmonary artery occlusion pressure (PAOP).
At that point, the doctor will deflate the balloon. Without the inflated balloon to support it, the catheter tip will slip back into the main branch of the pulmonary artery, making the PAP waveform reappear (see the waveform in Step 3). Now the catheter's placed correctly. The doctor will finish the procedure by securely suturing the catheter to the patient's skin.

PULMONARY ARTERY WEDGE
PRESSURE (P.A.W.P.)

Normal range
Mean: 8 to 12 mm Hg
4. Blood flow in the pulmonary artery will then carry the catheter balloon into one of the pulmonary artery's many smaller branches.

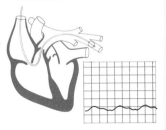

Troubleshooting Other Common Hemodynamic Pressure Monitoring Problems

PROBLEM/POSSIBLE CAUSES	NURSING ACTION

No waveform

• Power supply off	• Check power supply.
• Oscilloscope's pressure range set too low	• Reset oscilloscope's pressure range higher, if necessary. Then rebalance and recalibrate the equipment.
• Loose connection in line • Transducer's stopcock off to patient	• Tighten any loose connections and position stopcocks correctly.
• Catheter occluded or out of blood vessel	• Use fast flush valve to flush line. • Try to aspirate blood from the catheter. If the line still won't flush, notify the doctor and prepare to replace the line.

Drifting waveforms

• Monitor and transducer not warmed up properly	• Allow monitor and transducer to warm up 10 to 15 minutes.
• Monitor's electrical cable compressed	• Place monitor's cable where it can't be stepped on or compressed.
• Temperature change in room air or I.V. flush solution	• Remember to routinely rebalance and recalibrate 30 minutes after setting up the equipment. This gives the I.V. fluid sufficient time to warm to room temperature.

Continued

Troubleshooting Other Common Hemodynamic Pressure Monitoring Problems

Continued

PROBLEM/POSSIBLE CAUSES	NURSING ACTION
Line won't flush	
• Stopcock positioned incorrectly	• Check stopcocks to make sure they're positioned correctly.
• Inadequate pressure from pressure bag	• Check pressure bag to make sure pressure reads 300 mm Hg.
• Kink in pressure tubing or blood clot in catheter	• Check pressure tubing for kinks. • Try aspirating blood clot with a syringe. • If the line still won't flush, notify the doctor and prepare to replace the line. *Important:* Never use a syringe to flush any hemodynamic line.
Artifact (waveform interference)	
• Patient movement	• Wait until the patient's quiet before taking a reading.
• Catheter fling (tip of pulmonary artery [PA] catheter moving rapidly in large blood vessel or heart chamber)	• Notify the doctor of catheter fling. He may try to reposition the catheter.
• Electrical interference	• Make sure electrical equipment's connected and grounded correctly.

Continued

CARDIOVASCULAR CARE

Troubleshooting Other Common Hemodynamic Pressure Monitoring Problems
Continued

PROBLEM/POSSIBLE CAUSES	NURSING ACTION
False-high readings	
• Transducer's balancing port positioned below the patient's right atrium	• Position the transducer's balancing port level with the patient's right atrium.
• Transducer unbalanced	• Rebalance and recalibrate the equipment. • Check transducer's cable, and make sure it's not kinked or occluded.
• Flush solution flow rate too fast	• Check flow rate of flush solution. Maintain it at 3 to 4 ml per hour.
• Catheter fling	• Notify doctor of catheter fling. He may try to reposition the catheter.
False-low readings	
• Transducer's balancing port positioned above the patient's right atrium	• Position transducer's balancing port level with right atrium.
• Loose connection in line	• Check all connections and tighten them, if necessary.

CARDIOVASCULAR CARE

Troubleshooting a Damped Waveform

Normal pulmonary artery
pressure (PAP) waveform

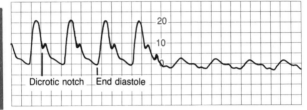

Normal pulmonary artery wedge
pressure (PAWP) waveform

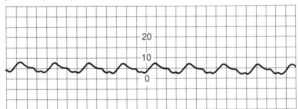

Continued

Troubleshooting a Damped Waveform
Continued

AIR BUBBLES SOME-
WHERE IN LINE; FOR EX-
AMPLE, TUBING,
TRANSDUCER DOME, OR
STOPCOCKS

Nursing action
• Check stopcocks and make
sure they're positioned correctly.
• Check the line for leaks.
Then, replace the line, if necessary.
• Check for loose connec-
tions, especially dome connections, and tighten them, if
necessary.
• Take care to flush out air
bubbles through an open
stopcock port.
Prevention
• Flush all air from line when
setting up equipment.
• Avoid rapid, repeated pulling of the pigtail on the fast
flush valve. This causes tur-
bulence in the flushing solution, which in turn produces
air bubbles.
• Make sure the drip chamber is at least half-full at all
times. Avoid use of microdrip
tubing.

BLOOD CLOT IN CATHETER
OR STOPCOCK

Nursing action
• Pull the pigtail on the fast
flush valve to flush catheter. *Important:* Never flush any hemo-
dynamic line with a syringe. You
may cause an embolus.
• Try to aspirate the clotted
blood with a syringe.
• If the catheter remains clotted, notify the doctor and prepare to replace the line.
Prevention
• Maintain adequate flow rate
of heparinized flush solution
(3 to 4 ml per hour).
• Use the fast flush valve to
flush the catheter after drawing blood samples.

ARTERIAL CATHETER
PULLED OUT OF BLOOD
VESSEL OR PRESSED
AGAINST VESSEL WALL

Nursing action
• Pull the pigtail on the fast
flush valve.

Continued

Troubleshooting a Damped Waveform
Continued

ARTERIAL CATHETER PULLED OUT OF BLOOD VESSEL OR PRESSED AGAINST VESSEL WALL
Continued

● Attempt to aspirate blood to confirm proper placement in vessel.
● If you can't aspirate blood, notify doctor and prepare to replace the line. *Note:* Bloody drainage at the insertion site may indicate catheter displacement. Notify the doctor at once.
Prevention
● Tape the catheter securely.
● Stabilize the insertion site with a splint.

PULMONARY ARTERY (P.A.) CATHETER PRESSED OR WEDGED AGAINST BLOOD VESSEL WALL

Nursing action
● Deflate balloon on PA catheter completely.
● Ask patient to cough. This may jolt the catheter free.
● Fast flush the catheter, us-

ing the fast flush valve. This also may jolt it free.
● Notify the doctor, so he can reposition the catheter, if necessary.
● Prepare the patient for a chest X-ray to confirm correct catheter placement.
Prevention
● Make sure the catheter is securely sutured and taped.
● Observe PA waveforms closely.
● Make sure the balloon's *completely* deflated after each use.

REGULAR I.V. TUBING USED BETWEEN CATHETER AND TRANSDUCER

Nursing action
● Replace I.V. tubing with rigid pressure tubing.
Prevention
● Always use rigid pressure tubing between the catheter and the transducer. Regular I.V. tubing expands under pressure, causing damped waveforms.

Continued

Troubleshooting a Damped Waveform
Continued

TRANSDUCER NOT BAL-
ANCED PROPERLY

Nursing action
• Check transducer cable for
occlusion or compression.
• Level the transducer's balancing port with the patient's
right atrium, and balance the
transducer to atmospheric
pressure.
• Recalibrate the monitor
with the transducer.
Prevention
• Keep transducer cable off
the floor so it isn't damaged.
• Reposition the transducer
whenever the patient's position changes. Remember, its
balancing port must always
be level with the patient's
right atrium.
• Rebalance and recalibrate
equipment if the room temperature changes signifi-
cantly.

• Rebalance and recalibrate
equipment routinely, at least
once every 8 hours.
Nursing tip: When using a
standard-sized transducer,
avoid putting more than two
or three drops of sterile water
between the transducer and
the dome. Too much fluid can
dampen the waveform.

BLOOD BACKUP IN LINE

Nursing action
• Check stopcock positions
and make sure they're correct.
• Check for loose connec-
tions and tighten them, if necessary.
• Use the fast flush valve to
flush blood from catheter.
• Replace dome if blood
backs up into it.
Prevention
• Maintain 300 mm Hg of
pressure in the pressure bag
at all times.

Some Cardiovascular Drugs

ATROPINE SULFATE

Use, route, and dosage
Anticholinergic (for bradycardia) — I.V. bolus 0.5 mg; may repeat
Side effects
Therapeutic dosages: dry mouth, cycloplegia, and mydriasis
Large dosages: hyperpyrexia, urinary retention, confusion, and hallucinations
Nursing tips
• When protocol allows, give to patients with bradycardia (rate < 50 BPM) who have hypotension, syncope, dyspnea, or ventricular dysrhythmias.

CLONIDINE HYDROCHLORIDE

Catapres*
Use, route, and dosage
Antihypertensive — P.O.: initial dose 0.1 mg b.i.d.; increase by 0.1 to 0.2 mg/day until desired response obtained; usual maintenance dose is 0.2 to 0.8 mg daily in divided doses
Side effects
Dry mouth, drowsiness, sedation, constipation, dizziness, headache, fatigue
Nursing tips
• Don't discontinue abruptly.
• Warn patient about sedative effect.
• Patient should not drink alcohol or take sedatives with this drug.

CALCIUM CHLORIDE

Use, route, and dosage
Cardiac stimulant — I.V. bolus, intracardiac 1 g (10 ml of a 10% solution); may repeat
Side effects
Cardiac dysrhythmia (in digitalized patients), venous irritation, vasodilation, hypotension, bradycardia, syncope, and cardiac arrest
Nursing tips
• Very irritating; take extreme care to avoid extravasation when giving I.V.
• Avoid using in digitalized patients; may cause fatal dysrhythmia.

DOPAMINE HYDROCHLORIDE

Intropin*
Use, route, and dosage
Adrenergic, inotropic agent — I.V. infusion 5 mcg/kg/min up to 50 mcg/kg/min
Side effects
Ectopic beats, tachycardia, angina, palpitation, vasoconstriction, hypotension, dyspnea, nausea and vomiting, and headache
Nursing tips
• Do not add to alkaline solutions; for example, sodium bicarbonate.
• Monitor EKG for ventricular dysrhythmias.
• Check urine output q 30 min.
Continued

Some Cardiovascular Drugs
Continued

DOPAMINE HYDROCHLORIDE
Continued

• Rate of infusion is adjusted according to cardiac output, peripheral perfusion, urine output, and pulmonary and arterial pressures; monitor all these parameters closely.
• Must be diluted to 250- to 500-ml volume before using.

DISOPYRAMIDE (BASE OR PHOSPHATE)

Norpace*
Rythmodan**
Use, route, and dosage
Antiarrhythmic — P.O.: loading dose 300 mg, then 100 to 150 mg q 6 hr
Side effects
Dry mouth, eyes, nose, throat; urinary hesitancy or retention; urinary frequency or urgency; GI distress; constipation; blurred vision; weight gain (edema); headache; generalized fatigue and weakness; dizziness; rash; nervousness; hypotension; shortness of breath; chest pain; and syncope
Nursing tips
• Don't give to patients in cardiogenic shock, second- or third-degree AV block.
• Give cautiously to patients with renal or liver disease.
  *Available in the United States and Canada.
**Available only in Canada.

• If hypotension or heart failure occurs, notify the doctor immediately.

EPINEPHRINE HYDROCHLORIDE

Adrenalin
Use, route, and dosage
Adrenergic, cardiac stimulant — I.V. bolus, intracardiac 0.5 to 1 mg (5 to 10 ml of 1:10,000 sol); may repeat
Side effects
Fear, anxiety, headache, tremor, dizziness, disorientation, nausea and vomiting, sweating, pallor, respiratory difficulty and apnea, palpitations, tachycardia, angina, ventricular dysrhythmias
Nursing tips
• Watch for pulmonary edema due to peripheral vasoconstriction.
• Stop if headache, chest pain, nausea, or hypotension occur.
• I.V. injection of 1:1,000 solution leads to hypertension, subarachnoid hemorrhage, and hemiplegia.

DIGOXIN

Lanoxin*
Use, route, and dosage
Congestive heart failure, atrial fibrillation and flutter, paroxysmal atrial tachycardia—Loading
Continued

Some Cardiovascular Drugs
Continued

DIGOXIN
Continued

dose: 0.5 to 1 mg I.V. or P.O. in divided doses over 24 hours; maintenance 0.125 to 0.5 mg I.V. or P.O. daily (average 0.25 mg; however, less in elderly patients and those with renal insufficiency); larger doses often needed for treatment of arrhythmias, depending on patient response

Side effects
Fatigue, generalized muscle weakness, agitation, hallucinations, headache, malaise, dizziness, vertigo, stupor, paresthesias, increased severity of congestive heart failure, arrhythmias, hypotension, yellow-green halos around visual images, blurred vision, light flashes, photophobia, diplopia, anorexia, nausea, vomiting, and diarrhea

Nursing tips
• Obtain baseline data before giving first dose.
• Monitor serum potassium carefully.
• Take apical-radial pulse for a full minute. Record and report to doctor any significant changes.

• Excessive slowing of pulse rate (60/min or less) may be sign of digoxin toxicity.
• Drug is contraindicated in presence of any digitalis-induced toxicity, ventricular fibrillation, or ventricular tachycardia, unless caused by congestive heart failure.
• Use cautiously in patients with acute myocardial infarction; incomplete AV block; chronic constrictive pericarditis; idiopathic hypertrophic subaortic stenosis; renal insufficiency; severe pulmonary disease; hypothyroidism; and in the elderly.

HYDRALAZINE HYDROCHLORIDE

Apresoline*
Rolazine
Use, route, and dosage
Afterload reducer, antihypertensive — P.O.: Initial dose 10 mg q.i.d. for 4 days, then 25 mg q.i.d. for 3 days, then 50 mg q.i.d. thereafter. Maintenance: lowest effective dose.
I.V., I.M.: 20 to 40 mg repeated as necessary
Side effects
Headache, palpitations, GI disturbance, tachycardia, angina, flushing, peripheral neuritis, edema, anxiety, lupus-like syndrome

Continued

Some Cardiovascular Drugs
Continued

HYDRALAZINE HYDROCHLO-RIDE
Continued

Nursing tips
• Watch for signs of myocardial ischemia; angina, and EKG changes.
• Use cautiously in patients with suspected coronary artery disease.

ISOPROTERENOL HYDRO-CHLORIDE

Isuprel*
Use, route, and dosage
Beta-adrenergic, cardiac stimulant—I.V. bolus, intracardiac 0.02 mg; I.V. infusion of 1 mg/500 ml D_5W titrated to heart rate and blood pressure
Side effects
Arrhythmias, palpitations, tachycardia, headache, flushing, dizziness, sweating, and tremors
Nursing tips
• Slow or stop infusion if heart rate exceeds 110/min.
• Discontinue if ventricular arrhythmia occurs.
• Have defibrillator at bedside.
• Measure urine output and B.P. every 15 min.

• Do not use concurrently with epinephrine; may cause serious arrhythmias.

LIDOCAINE HYDROCHLORIDE

Xylocaine*
Use, route, and dosage
Ventricular antiarrhythmic —
I.V. bolus 100 mg followed by I.V. infusion 1 to 2 g/500 ml D_5W at 1 to 4 mg/min; may repeat bolus q 3 to 5 min. Don't exceed 300 mg total bolus during 1 hr.
Side effects
Hypotension, cardiovascular collapse, bradycardia, convulsions, respiratory depression, visual disturbances, and slurred speech. Severe reactions may be preceded by somnolence and paresthesia.
Nursing tips
• Give cautiously to patients with Stokes-Adams syndrome, liver disease, or CHF; may cause toxicity.
• If CNS side effects occur, stop the infusion immediately, give O_2, and call the doctor.

Continued

*Available in the United States and Canada.
**Available only in Canada.

Some Cardiovascular Drugs
Continued

CARDIOVASCULAR CARE

METARAMINOL BITARTRATE

Aramine
Use, route, and dosage
Alpha- and beta-adrenergic, vasopressor —I.V. 15 to 100 mg/500 ml D$_5$NS. Adjust rate to maintain B.P.
Side effects
Anxiety, tremor, faintness, headache, dizziness, precordial pain, respiratory difficulty, flushing, pallor, sweating, and nausea
Nursing tips
• Monitor vital signs q 30 min.
• MAO inhibitors potentiate its pressor effect.
• Guanethidine-metaraminol interaction may cause hypertensive crisis.

METHYLDOPA

Aldomet*
Use, route, and dosage
Antihypertensive — P.O.: Initial dose 250 mg b.i.d. or t.i.d. for 2 days, then increase or decrease dose every 2 days until desired effect obtained.
Maintenance: 500 mg to 3 g daily in 2 to 4 doses.
I.V. infusion: 250 to 500 mg (maximum dose 1g) in 100 ml D$_5$W over 30 to 60 min q 6 hr (dose titrated according to B.P.)

Side effects
Sedation, headache, and weakness (all transient); orthostatic hypotension; edema; GI distress; liver function test abnormalities; positive Coombs' test; drug fever; rash; impotence; dry mouth; and nasal stuffiness
Nursing tips
• Use cautiously in patients with liver disease.
• Warn patients about sedative effect.
• Baseline blood count recommended at start and periodically during therapy.

NITROPRUSSIDE SODIUM

Nipride*
Use, route, and dosage
Vasodilator, antihypertensive — I.V. 0.5 to 10 mcg/kg/min continuous I.V. infusion. Use only D$_5$W for dilution; to make solution containing 100 mcg/ml, dilute 50 mg nitroprusside in 500 ml D$_5$W
Side effects
GI disturbance, increased perspiration, headache, restlessness, apprehension, muscle twitching, retrosternal discomfort, palpitations, dizziness, hypotension, and irritation at infusion site

Continued

Some Cardiovascular Drugs
Continued

NITROPRUSSIDE SODIUM
Continued

Nursing tips
• Protect container from light — wrap in foil.
• Prepare fresh infusion q 4 hr.
• Use infusion pump.
• Avoid extravasation.
• Monitor vital signs q 5 min while the infusion is being started, then q 15 min.
• Discard solution after 24 hr.

NOREPINEPHRINE INJECTION (FORMERLY LEVARTERENOL BITARTRATE)

Levophed*
Use, route, and dosage
Alpha- and beta-adrenergic, vasopressor—I.V. infusion 8 to 16 mg (2 to 4 amps) in 500 ml D_5W titrated to blood pressure
Side effects
Intense sweating, vomiting, severe hypertension, headache, weakness, dizziness, tremor, pallor, respiratory difficulty, precordial pain, cardiac arrhythmias, and tissue necrosis and sloughing from extravasation of injection
Nursing tips
• Check infusion site frequently to avoid extravasation. Should extravasation occur, stop infusion and flush the area immediately with 15 ml of saline solution and 10 ml of phentolamine to avoid sloughing of tissue.
• Guanethidine and methyldopa increase norepinephrine's effect.

PRAZOSIN HYDROCHLORIDE

Minipress*
Use, route and dosage
Vasodilator, antihypertensive — P.O.: Initial dose 1 mg t.i.d. Maintenance: 3 to 20 mg daily in divided doses (a few patients may require up to 40 mg daily)
Side effects
Severe syncope may occur if initial dose greater than 1 mg; headache, drowsiness, weakness, palpitations, GI disturbance, edema, dry mouth, and dizziness
Nursing tips
• Observe closely for syncopal episodes after initial dose and each dosage increase. Such episodes usually occur within 60 to 90 min after dose.
• Administer initial dose at bedtime to minimize effect of syncope.

Continued

*Available in the United States and Canada.
**Available only in Canada.

CARDIOVASCULAR CARE

Some Cardiovascular Drugs
Continued

CARDIOVASCULAR CARE

PROCAINAMIDE HYDROCHLORIDE

Pronestyl*
Use, route, and dosage
Ventricular antiarrhythmic —
P.O.: 250 to 500 mg q 3 to 4 hr
I.M.: 0.5 to 1 g q 6 hr until patient can take drug P.O.
I.V.: 100 mg q 5 min (at rate of 20 to 50 mg/min) up to maximum loading dose of 1g or until dysrhythmia is suppressed. Drip of 2 to 6 mg/min may be used after loading dose.
Side effects
Hypotension and serious disturbances of cardiac rhythm due to Q-T prolongation with I.M. or I.V. routes, GI disturbances, urticaria, pruritus, fever, chills, weakness, depression, psychosis, lupus-like syndrome and positive antinuclear antigen test (during prolonged therapy), and agranulocytosis
Nursing tips
• Watch for cardiac dysrhythmias, atrial fibrillation, and ventricular tachycardia after I.V. administration.
• Tell patient to report any sore throat or sores in mouth, unexplained fever, or upper respiratory tract infection.
• Use I.V. route only for emergencies.

PROPRANOLOL HYDROCHLORIDE

Inderal*
Inderal LA*
Use, route, and dosage
Antihypertensive, antianginal, antiarrhythmic—P.O.: Hypertension, 80 to 640 mg daily in divided doses; or sustained-release capsule once daily. Angina and dysrhythmias, 10 to 40 mg q.i.d.
I.V.: 1 to 3 mg
Side effects
Bradycardia, CHF, intensification of AV block, hypotension, lightheadedness, visual disturbances, GI distress, bronchospasm; exacerbation of angina and MI may follow abrupt withdrawal of drug; and mental disturbances ranging from disorientation to catatonia
Nursing tips
• Do not discontinue abruptly.
• Note small I.V. dose compared to P.O. dose.
• Use I.V. route only for life-threatening arrhythmias.
• Drug may mask signs of hypoglycemia in diabetic patients.

Continued

Some Cardiovascular Drugs
Continued

QUINIDINE GLUCONATE
Duraquin, Quinaglute Dura-Tabs*,
Quinate**
QUINIDINE POLYGALACTURON-
ATE
Cardioquin*
QUINIDINE SULFATE
CinQuin, Quine, Quinidex Extentabs, Quinora, SK-Quinidine Sulfate

Use, route, and dosage
Atrial and ventricular antiarrhythmic—P.O.: 200 to 400 mg q 4 to 6 hr
I.M.: Initial dose 300 to 400 mg
then 200 mg q 2 hr times four (for
acute tachycardia)
Side effects
Tinnitus, headache, disturbed vision, cardiac asystole, ventricular
dysrhythmias, widening of QRS
complex, paradoxical tachycardia,
GI disturbance, vertigo, excitement,
confusion, cutaneous flushing with
intense pruritus, hypersensitivity reaction, and fever
Nursing tips
• Give test dose (200 mg) to determine idiosyncrasy; observe patient closely; take vital signs
frequently.

• Give cautiously to patients in incomplete AV block (may cause
complete AV block).
• Widening of QRS complex by
50% is sign of quinidine cardiotoxicity. Stop drug immediately.

RESERPINE
Serpasil*
Reserpanca**

Use, route, and dosage
Antihypertensive—P.O.: Initial
dose 0.5 mg daily for 1 to 2
weeks.
Maintenance 0.1 to 0.5 mg daily.
I.M.: Initial dose 0.5 to 1 mg, then
2 to 4 mg q 3 hr until desired response
Side effects
Depression, GI disturbances including hypersecretion, anginalike symptoms, dysrhythmias,
drowsiness, nervousness, anxiety,
nightmares, dull sensorium, deafness, nasal congestion, pruritus,
rash, dry mouth, dizziness, headache, impotence, dysuria, myalgias, and edema
Nursing tips
• Use cautiously in patients with
renal disease (lowered B.P. may further compromise renal function).

Continued

Some Cardiovascular Drugs
Continued

RESERPINE
Continued

• Avoid in patients with history of mental depression.
• Watch closely for signs of developing despondency.
• Contraindicated in patients with ulcer disease or ulcerative colitis.

SODIUM BICARBONATE

Use, route, and dosage
To prevent acidosis—I.V. bolus 1 mEq/kg; repeat in 10 min, if necessary. Further doses based on blood gas analysis. If ABGs unavailable, use 0.5 mEq/kg every 10 min. during resuscitation.
Side effects
Metabolic alkalosis
Nursing tips
• Incompatible with calcium solutions.
• A 4.2% solution, slow administration, is preferred for children under age 2.
• Watch for signs of alkalosis: nausea, vomiting, diarrhea, slow and shallow respirations, confusion, irritability, and twitching.

VERAPAMIL

Use, route, and dosage
Calcium channel blocker, antiarrhythmic—I.V. push 0.075 to 0.15 mg/kg (5 to 10 mg) over 60 seconds with EKG and blood pressure monitoring. Repeat dose in 30 minutes if no response. Follow bolus injection with maintenance infusion of 0.005 mg/kg/min.
Side effects
Dizziness, headache, transient hypotension, heart failure, bradycardia, AV block, ventricular systole, and constipation
Nursing tips
• Give cautiously to patients with myocardial infarction followed by coronary occlusion, sick sinus syndrome, impaired AV conduction, and heart failure with atrial tachydysrhythmia.
• Note that patients with severely compromised cardiac function or those receiving beta blockers should receive lower doses.
• Contraindicated in patients with advanced heart failure, AV block, cardiogenic shock, sinus node disease, and severe hypotension.
• Drug should not be given within 30 minutes if patient received I.V. beta blocker; both cause myocardial depression.

Highlighting Streptokinase

If streptokinase is given to a patient with an acute myocardial infarction, his chances of survival and recovery may improve. Here's why:

Streptokinase is a thrombolytic, so it dissolves the clot occluding the artery. This improves myocardial perfusion and, if the drug's given within 3 to 4 hours of the onset of the patient's chest pain, it limits the infarction's size.

Administering streptokinase directly into the occluded coronary artery, using angiography in a cardiac catheterization laboratory, is the most effective treatment. (You may also give streptokinase by continuous I.V. for such disorders as pulmonary emboli and deep-vein thrombosis.)

Remember these important points about administering streptokinase:
• Always establish a perfusion baseline of peripheral pulses.
• Before infusion, double-check all doses and infusion rates with another nurse.
• Don't give intramuscular or intravenous injections during infusion or for 24 hours afterward.
• Establish two I.V. lines before infusion. Use one for streptokinase, the second for any other drugs you need to give.
• Align and immobilize the affected limb.
• Inspect the infusion site hourly for signs of bleeding. After infusion, inspect the site every 15 minutes the first hour, every 30 minutes for 2 to 8 hours, then once per shift.
• Monitor and document the following every hour, before and after infusion: the patient's pulses and color, and the sensitivity of his affected and unaffected limbs.
• Keep a laboratory flow sheet so you can monitor the following during and after infusion: partial thromboplastin time, prothrombin time, hemoglobin, and hematocrit.
• Monitor carefully, for dysrhythmias, any patient receiving intracoronary streptokinase for lysis of coronary artery thrombi.
• Test all the patient's nasogastric aspirate and his stools and urine for blood, during and after infusion.
• Apply direct pressure to the infusion site for at least 30 minutes after the catheter's removed.
• Watch the patient for flushing, itching, urticaria, headaches and muscle aches, and nausea. These may indicate a mild allergic and febrile reaction.

Guide to Some Drugs That Affect the Cardiovascular System

CLASSIFICATION	POSSIBLE SIDE EFFECTS
Anticonvulsants diazepam (Valium*)	• Hypotension, bradycardia, cardiovascular collapse
phenytoin sodium (Dilantin*)	• Hypotension, ventricular fibrillation, nystagmus, ataxia, diplopia, blurred vision
Antidepressants amitriptyline hydrochloride (Elavil*) doxepin hydrochloride (Sinequan*)	• Orthostatic hypotension, tachycardia, EKG changes, hypertension
Antipsychotics chlorpromazine hydrochloride (Thorazine) thioridazine (Mellaril*)	• Orthostatic hypotension, tachycardia, dysrhythmias
Cerebral stimulants amphetamine sulfate (Benzedrine*)	• Tachycardia, palpitations, hypertension, hypotension
caffeine (Nodoz, Vivarin)	• Tachycardia
Cholinergics (parasympathomimetics) bethanechol chloride (Urecholine*)	• Bradycardia, hypotension, cardiac arrest, tachycardia

Continued

CARDIOVASCULAR CARE

Guide to Some Drugs That Affect the Cardiovascular System
Continued

CLASSIFICATION	POSSIBLE SIDE EFFECTS
Estrogens chlorotrianisene (Tace*) esterified estrogens (Amnestrogen, Climestrone**)	• Thrombophlebitis, thromboembolism, hypertension, edema, risk of cerebrovascular accident, pulmonary embolism, myocardial infarction
Nonnarcotic analgesics and antipyretics indomethacin (Indocid**, Indocin)	• Hypertension, edema
phenylbutazone (Butazolidin*)	• Hypertension, pericarditis, myocarditis, cardiac decompensation
Oral contraceptives estrogen with progestogen (Demulen*)	• Thromboembolism, thrombophlebitis, hypertension
Sedatives and hypnotics ethchlorvynol (Placidyl*) paraldehyde (Paral)	• Hypotension • By I.V. administration: pulmonary edema, hemorrhage, right-sided heart failure
Spasmolytics aminophylline (Aminophyllin)	• Sinus tachycardia, extrasystoles, flushing, hypotension

*Available in the United States and Canada.
**Available only in Canada.

Troubleshooting Pacemaker Problems

CARDIOVASCULAR CARE

FAILURE TO CAPTURE

(Pacemaker transmits impulses to heart but fails to stimulate it)

Signs
• Apical rate is below pacemaker setting.
• Pacemaker spike is not followed by QRS complex on EKG.
• Continuous sense/pace dial movement.

Possible causes
• Dislodged catheter
• Pacemaker end-of-life or premature battery depletion
• Fractured lead wire
• Change in output threshold (stimulation threshold)

Possible solutions
• Turn patient on left side to aid catheter contact with myocardium.
• Replace the battery.
• Lead wire replaced by doctor.
• Notify doctor and monitor patient closely. Doctor may increase output threshold or reposition catheter. (*Note:* In some institutions, nurse may increase stimulation threshold to reestablish capture before calling doctor.)

FAILURE TO SENSE

(pacemaker fails to detect ventricular depolarization and functions independently of heart rate)

Signs
• Apical rate is higher than pacemaker setting and irregular.
• Pacemaker beats follow normal beats at a rate higher than pacemaker setting.
• Continuous sense/pacer dial movement.

Possible causes
• Mode dial accidentally set at *fixed* mode.
• Dislodged catheter
• Competition between pacemaker's rhythm and patient's rhythm possibly resulting in ventricular fibrillation

Possible solutions
• Turn the dial to *demand* mode.
• See "Failure to capture."
• Turn the pacemaker off. Call the doctor to reposition the catheter. Monitor the patient closely to make sure his heart rate can maintain adequate cardiac output.

FIRING LOSS

(combined failure to sense/capture caused by mechanical failure of the unit)

Signs
• No pacing seen
• No sense/pace dial movement

Possible causes
• Dislodged catheter
• Pacemaker accidentally turned off

Continued

Troubleshooting Pacemaker Problems
Continued

FIRING LOSS
Continued

- Battery failure
- Loose catheter terminals
- Pacemaker generator worn out
- Broken catheter wires

Possible solutions
- See "Failure to capture."
- Turn the pacemaker on.
- Replace the battery.

- Tighten the terminals, wearing rubber gloves to avoid risk of electric shock for patient.
- Replace generator. Monitor patient's apical rate and blood pressure until pacemaker functions correctly.
- Catheter wires replaced by the doctor. Monitor the patient closely.

Special Consideration

Watch for signs of pacemaker malfunction. Make sure all electrical equipment is grounded with three-pronged plugs inserted in the right receptacles. *This protects the patient from accidental shocks to the heart that may cause ventricular fibrillation.* Also, cover all exposed metal parts of the pacemaker setup, such as electrode connections or pacemaker terminals, with nonconductive tape, or place the pacing unit in a dry rubber surgical glove, *to insulate it.* Instruct the patient not to use an electric razor or any other nonessential electrical equipment.

If emergency defibrillation should be necessary, make sure the pacemaker can withstand this procedure before starting it; if not, disconnect it *to avoid damaging the generator.*

Protect the pacemaker and its connections from moisture.

If the patient is disoriented or uncooperative, restrain his arms to prevent accidental removal of pacemaker wires.

If any evidence of infection is present during catheter implantation, culture disposable pacemaker catheter tips after they're removed.

Pacemaker Tips

- Explain to the patient why the procedure is necessary and how it will be performed.
- Show the patient a pacemaker; explain how it works.
- Watch him carefully after insertion to verify that the pacemaker is functioning properly and effectively.
- Watch for loss of capture, competition, signs of perforation, thrombophlebitis, or skin infection.
- Tell the patient and his family at what rate his pacemaker is set.

TEMPORARY PACEMAKER

- After the electrode has been introduced, gradually turn the energy control dial clockwise until you note a QRS complex with each stimulus. This is the patient's threshold level (usually about 1.5 milliamperes). As a safety precaution, this number is usually doubled to assure continued pacing.
- If loss of capture occurs:

change the patient's position, the battery, or the pacemaker unit. Notify the doctor.
- When discontinuing the pacemaker, turn the rate down *gradually* to avoid causing asystole.

PERMANENT PACEMAKER

- Teach the patient and family how to count and record his pulse daily.
- Explain the signs of battery failure: change in pacing rate, dizziness, Stokes-Adams attacks, dyspnea, or increased weight gain.
- Have the patient watch for signs of infection or skin breakdown.
- Tell him when to notify the doctor: when his pulse rate changes or symptoms recur; he has signs of infection; or he has suffered a blow that may have damaged his pacemaker.
- Make sure the patient understands the necessity of follow-up care at regular intervals.

Keeping Pace

Temporary transvenous pacemakers are usually inserted via the subclavian or external jugular veins or a cutdown in the arm. With a fluoroscope the doctor threads the catheter through the vein to the right ventricle. The

most common site for permanent pacemaker implantation is a pocket the doctor forms in the right anterior chest. From here he threads the catheter through a vein—most commonly the right cephalic—into the right ventricle.

Signs of Increased Intracranial Pressure

Increased intracranial pressure results from an increase in the volume of one or more intracranial components (brain tissue, blood, cerebrospinal fluid [CSF]) that exceeds the brain's compensatory capacity. Its severity depends on the size and rate of the volume increase, the total volume of the intracranial vault, and the relative volumes of other intracranial components available for displacement. Causes of increased intracranial pressure include hemorrhage, edema, hyperemia, impaired autoregulation, and hydrocephalus.

- Deteriorating level of consciousness

- Pupillary dilation (especially unilateral)

- Decreased pupillary light reflex

- Loss of motor function

- Sensory deterioration

- Rising systolic blood pressure

- Bradycardia

- Respiratory pattern changes

- Papilledema

- Headache

- Vomiting

Recognizing Abnormal Postures

A patient exhibiting any of the three abnormal postures described here may have severe neurologic damage. If your patient assumes any of these postures, alert the doctor immediately.

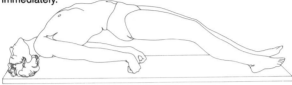

Opisthotonos: characterized by a rigidly arched neck and spine; may indicate meningeal irritation or seizures.

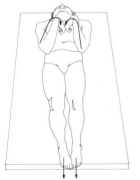

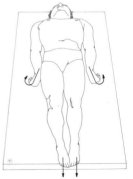

Decorticate posturing: a rigid spine, inwardly flexed arms, extended legs, and plantar flexion; may indicate a lesion at the level of the diencephalon.

Decerebrate posturing: a rigid and possibly arched spine, rigidly extended arms and legs, and plantar flexion; may indicate a brain stem lesion.

NEUROLOGIC CARE

The Neurologic Check

The chart below shows the changes in mental state, pupil dilation, and vital signs that accompany a fatal increase of intracranial pressure.

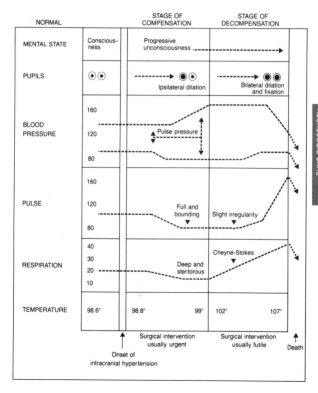

Intracranial Pressure (ICP) Monitoring

Monitoring can detect elevated intracranial pressure (ICP) early, before clinical danger signs develop. Prompt intervention can then help avert or diminish neurologic damage caused by cerebral hypoxia and shifts of brain mass.

The three basic ICP monitoring systems use a ventricular catheter, subarachnoid screw, or epidural sensor. Regardless of the devices used, this procedure is always performed by a neurosurgeon in the operating room, emergency room, or critical care unit. Insertion of an ICP monitoring device requires sterile technique to reduce the risk of CNS infection. Setting up equipment for the monitoring systems also requires strict asepsis.

Contraindications to ventricular catheter ICP monitoring usually include stenotic cerebral ventricles, cerebral aneurysms in the path of catheter placement, and suspected vascular lesions.

Calibrating an ICP Monitor

To calibrate an intracranial pressure (ICP) monitor using the *cal factor,* first see if the cal factor is marked on the transducer. If not, obtain it by testing the transducer with a mercury sphygmomanometer, as the operator's manual directs. Depress the "balance" button. If the transducer is balanced properly, you'll get a zero reading. Release the button. Then, depress the "calibrate" button and, while holding this button down, use a screwdriver to turn the screw next to it until the digital reading equals the cal factor.

To use the *electric cal,* depress the "zero" button on the monitor. Make sure the digital readout is zero and the oscilloscope line is at zero. Then depress the "test/cal" button and turn the "sensitivity" knob until the digital reading is 100 mm Hg and the line runs on the 100 mm Hg level.

To use the *pre-cal,* simply test the function of the monitor and transducer, because they're already calibrated with each other. Depress the "test" button and "zero" button simultaneously and hold them. The digital reading will be zero and the oscilloscope line will be at zero if the equipment's working properly.

Balance and calibrate the transducer and monitor at least once every 4 hours.

Interpreting ICP Waveforms

As the illustration on the next page shows, the horizontal axis measures time (usually in minutes); the vertical axis measures intracranial pressure (in millimeters of mercury). When observing actual waveforms on the monitor, pay extra attention to amount and duration of pressure elevations.

Normal pressure. 0 to 10 mm Hg with an upper limit of 15 mm Hg is considered normal intracranial pressure. Remember, however, that ICP is not static and that elevation in itself is not detrimental. Everyday activity requiring Valsalva's maneuver can raise ICP as high as 100 mm Hg.

Three types of ICP waveforms: Figure 1. Plateau or "A" waves indicate rapid increases in pressure to 50 to 100 mm Hg. They are *sustained* elevations lasting approximately 5 to 20 minutes and followed by a rapid decrease in pressure. Patients who already have an elevated ICP are more likely to develop them. *Plateau waves may indicate ICP decompensation. Report them to the*

doctor immediately. Remember, the prognosis is usually grave for patients who sustain ICPs greater than 50 mm Hg for more than 20 minutes.

Figure 2. "B" waves. Peaked, sharp, rhythmic oscillations with a sawtooth pattern, thought to be related to changes in respiration. They occur every ½ to 2 minutes. Pressure may increase as much as 50 mm Hg, but elevations are *not sustained.* B waves are not clinically significant, and you don't have to notify the doctor.

Figure 3. "C" waves, correlated to changes in blood pressure, take the form of smaller rhythmic oscillations. Although they also may reach abnormal levels, they are not sustained elevations. C waves are not clinically significant, and you don't have to report them to the doctor.

Nursing Tip: Whenever you perform a nursing measure that may increase ICP, such as suctioning, make sure that you mark the readout strip or document such care in your nurse's notes.

Continued

NEUROLOGIC CARE

Interpreting ICP Waveforms
Continued

FIGURE 1

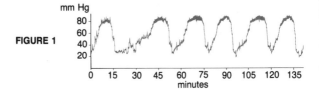

FIGURE 2

FIGURE 3

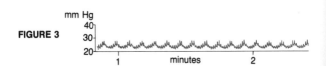

NEUROLOGIC CARE

Caring for the Patient with Elevated ICP

Does your patient have increased intracranial pressure (ICP)? Many procedures—even routine ones—tend to raise a patient's ICP. A cluster of nursing procedures done all at once may dangerously spike his ICP. So do your best to schedule stressful procedures separately. This chart will show you how to minimize or avoid other harmful stresses.

Note: The doctor may decide to monitor your patient's ICP with an invasive intracranial monitoring system.

MAINTAIN OXYGENATION; AVOID HYPOXIA AND/OR HYPERCAPNIA

Rationale
• A CO_2 excess and/or O_2 deficit in arterial blood stimulates cerebral vasodilation, increasing cerebral blood flow (CBF).
• Increasing CBF raises ICP.
Additional considerations
• Maintain a patent airway.
• Monitor arterial blood gas (ABG) measurements closely.
• Hyperventilate the patient before suctioning, to minimize CO_2 accumulation during the procedure.
• Limit suctioning to 10 to 15 seconds.

MAINTAIN VENOUS OUT-FLOW FROM THE BRAIN

Rationale
• Obstructions to venous outflow increase capillary pressure and diminish absorption of cerebrospinal fluid (CSF).
• Decreased outflow permits CO_2 and lactic acid to accumulate in the brain. Both stimulate cerebral vasodilation.
• ICP rises when venous outflow slows.
• As a response to rising ICP, blood pressure may drop, causing cerebral ischemia.
Additional considerations
• Do not place patient flat or in Trendelenburg position, unless ordered. Instead, elevate the patient's head 30°, or as ordered.
• Position the patient's head and neck directly above his midline to avoid compressing a jugular vein.
• If the patient has an endotracheal tube in place, make sure the tape securing it doesn't compress the jugular veins.

Continued

NEUROLOGIC CARE

Caring for the Patient with Elevated ICP
Continued

NEUROLOGIC CARE

AVOID INCREASING INTRA-THORACIC OR INTRA-ABDOMINAL PRESSURE

Rationale
• Added thoracic or abdominal pressure can spike ICP by increasing pressure on central veins.
Additional considerations
• Do not place patient in Trendelenburg position, even for insertion of jugular or subclavian vein catheter, unless the doctor orders.
• Do not ask the patient to execute Valsalva's maneuver, even during insertion of jugular or subclavian vein catheter. Instead, expect the doctor to minimize the danger of air embolism by using a syringe to apply suction to the catheter.
• Do your best to prevent the patient from using Valsalva's maneuver during bowel movements. Keep his stools soft with an appropriate diet and/or stool softeners. However, do not administer an enema.

• Prevent isometric muscular contractions. Assist your patient when he sits up, and instruct him not to push against the bed's footboard. But if the doctor orders, you may perform passive range-of-motion (ROM) exercises for the patient.
• Ask the patient to exhale when you turn him.
• Avoid hip flexion.

PREVENT WIDE OR SUDDEN VARIATIONS IN SYSTEMIC BLOOD PRESSURE

Rationale
• Normally autoregulation maintains cerebral perfusion pressure (CPP) at a level equal to mean systemic arterial pressure (MSAP) minus ICP. But autoregulation may fail when ICP is high. If so, CPP fluctuates with systemic blood pressure. Thus, an increase in systemic arterial pressure (SAP) increases cerebral blood flow (CBF), elevates ICP, and worsens cerebral edema.

Continued

Caring for the Patient with Elevated ICP
Continued

PREVENT WIDE OR SUDDEN VARIATIONS IN SYSTEMIC BLOOD PRESSURE
Continued

• Conversely, decreases in SAP may produce cerebral ischemia, allowing CO_2 and lactic acid to accumulate.

Additional considerations
• Use blood pressure and ICP monitors to evaluate the effect of stressful nursing procedures; for example, endotracheal tube insertion, suctioning, chest physiotherapy, and repositioning. Document your findings carefully.

• Minimize pain with a sedative or topical anesthetic, as ordered by the doctor.

• If ordered, use muscle relaxants to calm a combative patient during procedures like endotracheal tube insertion. However, avoid using restraints, unless ordered by the doctor.

• Rapid-eye-movement (REM) stages of sleep may cause a rise in ICP. Never perform stress-producing procedures during REM sleep.

PREVENT SYSTEMIC INFECTION (SEPSIS)

Rationale
• Systemic infection may produce increased cardiac output and vasodilation, increasing CBF.

Additional considerations
• Notify doctor promptly if the patient's temperature increases.

• If the patient's undergoing ICP monitoring, change the tubing and the dressing on the insertion site daily.

• Maintain scrupulous aseptic technique when changing any equipment or dressing.

• If the patient has a ventricular catheter in place, obtain a CSF sample daily, and send it to the lab for culturing. *Note:* Before obtaining a CSF sample from the drainage bag, remove the bag and tubing and replace them with sterile ones. Never open the CSF drainage bag while it's attached to the patient, or you risk infecting him.

NEUROLOGIC CARE

Anticonvulsants

DIAZEPAM

For status epilepticus: 5 to 20 mg by slow I.V. push; may repeat q 5 to 10 minutes to maximum dose of 60 mg

Interactions
None significant.

Side effects
Cardiovascular collapse, drowsiness, ataxia, pain at injection site, thrombophlebitis

Special considerations
• Contraindicated in shock, psychosis, coma, acute alcohol intoxication with depression of vital signs, acute narrow-angle glaucoma.
• Don't mix with other drugs or I.V. fluids. Avoid storing in plastic syringe or infusing through plastic tubing. Infuse at rate not exceeding 5 mg/minute and preferably at 2 mg/minute to decrease risk of respiratory depression and hypotension. Monitor respirations every 5 to 15 minutes and before each repeated dose. Have emergency resuscitative equipment and oxygen at bedside. Also watch for phlebitis at injection site.

PARALDEHYDE

For status epilepticus: 5 to 10 ml I.M.; 0.2 to 0.4 ml/kg in 0.9% saline by I.V. injection

Interactions
Alcohol: increased CNS depression. Use together cautiously.
Disulfiram: increased paraldehyde blood levels; possible toxic disulfiram reaction. Use together cautiously.

Side effects
Pulmonary edema or hemorrhage, circulatory collapse (from I.V. use), foul breath, odor, skin rash

Special considerations
• Contraindicated in gastroenteritis with ulceration. Use cautiously in impaired hepatic function or in asthma or other pulmonary disease.
• Divide 10 ml I.M. dose into two injections. Inject deeply, away from nerve trunks, and massage injection site. Use glass syringe and bottle for parenteral dose since drug reacts with plastic. Don't use if solution is brown or has a vinegary odor, or if container has been open longer than 24 hours.

Continued

Anticonvulsants
Continued

PHENOBARBITAL

For status epilepticus: 10 mg/kg by I.V. infusion no faster than 50 mg/minute; maximum dose—20 mg/kg
For epilepsy: usual maintenance dose—100 to 200 mg P.O. daily in single or divided doses

Interactions
Alcohol and other CNS depressants, including narcotic analgesics: excessive CNS depression.
MAO inhibitors: potentiated barbiturate effect.
Oral anticoagulants: possible decreased anticoagulant effect.
Rifampin: may decrease barbiturate levels. Monitor for decreased effect.

Side effects
Lethargy, drowsiness, hangover, skin eruptions

Special considerations
• Reserve I.V. injection for emergency treatment, and give slowly under close supervision. Monitor respirations carefully. Watch for signs of barbiturate toxicity; asthmatic breathing, cyanosis, clammy skin, hypotension, coma. Overdose can be fatal.
• Don't use injection solution if it contains a precipitate.

PHENYTOIN

For status epilepticus: 500 mg to 1 g I.V. at 50 mg/minute.
For epilepsy: maintenance dose—300 to 600 mg P.O. daily or in divided doses

Interactions
Alcohol, folic acid, loxapine: decreased phenytoin activity.
Oral anticoagulants, antihistamines, chloramphenicol, cimetidine, diazepam, diazoxide, disulfiram, isoniazid, phenylbutazone, salicylates, thioridazine, valproate: phenytoin toxicity risk.

Side effects
Nausea, vomiting, gingival hyperplasia, blood dyscrasias, rash, exfoliative dermatitis, hirsutism, nystagmus, diplopia, blurred vision, drowsiness, dizziness, confusion, hallucinations, slurred speech

Special considerations
• Give divided doses with or after meals to decrease GI side effects. Stop drug if skin rash appears. If rash is scarlet or measles-like, resume drug after rash clears. If rash reappears, stop drug. If rash is exfoliative, purpuric, or bullous, don't resume drug. Provide patient with instructions.
• Use only clear solution for injection. Consider slight yellowing acceptable. Don't refrigerate drug.

NEUROLOGIC CARE

Miscellaneous Drugs

DEXAMETHASONE

For cerebral edema: 10 mg I.V., then 4 to 6 mg I.M. q 6 hours for 2 to 4 days; then decrease dose over 5 to 7 days
Interactions
Indomethacin, aspirin: increased risk of GI distress and bleeding. Use together cautiously.
Side effects
Atrophy at I.M. injection sites, euphoria, insomnia, peptic ulcer
Special considerations
● Give I.M. injection deep into gluteal muscle. Avoid S.C. injections. When possible, replace I.M. with P.O. route.

LACTULOSE

For hepatic coma: 20 to 30 g (30 to 45 ml) P.O. t.i.d. or q.i.d. until patient has two or three soft stools daily
Interactions
None significant.
Side effects
Cramps, belching, flatulence, diarrhea, hypernatremia

Special considerations
● You can minimize drug's sweet taste with water, fruit juice, or food. Reduce dosage if diarrhea occurs. Replace fluid loss. Monitor serum sodium for hypernatremia, especially with high doses.

NEOMYCIN

For hepatic coma: 1 to 3 g P.O. q.i.d. for 5 to 6 days
Interactions
Dimenhydrinate: may mask symptoms of ototoxicity.
Ethacrynic acid, furosemide: increased ototoxicity.
Other aminoglycosides, methoxyflurane: increase ototoxicity and nephrotoxicity.
Side effects
Ototoxicity, nephrotoxicity
Special considerations
● Drug isn't absorbed at recommended dosage. However, more than 4 g of neomycin daily may be systemically absorbed and may lead to nephrotoxicity. Monitor renal function (urine output, specific gravity, BUN and creatinine levels, and creatinine clearance). Notify doctor of signs of decreasing renal function.

Hypovolemia: Recognizing Causes

What causes hypovolemia? Any condition that causes either external or internal fluid loss.

Carefully monitor your patient for early signs of hypovolemia if he has one of these diseases or conditions:
• External hemorrhage
• Internal hemorrhage (gastrointestinal bleeding, for example)
• Burns

• Trauma (such as fractures, gunshot wounds, or surgery)
• Bowel obstruction
• Peritonitis
• Diabetes insipidus
• Diabetic ketoacidosis
• Prolonged vomiting or diarrhea
• Inadequate fluid intake
• Excessive perspiration without fluid replacement
• Excessive diuretic use.

Checking for Hypovolemic Shock

Your chest trauma patient's skin is cool and clammy. He's restless and slightly tachypneic. You realize that these nonspecific symptoms may be caused by the transient stress of injury. But you should be concerned that hypovolemic shock may be the cause. This condition, which follows massive blood loss, may lead to irreversible cerebral and renal damage, cardiac arrest, and death. How can you determine whether your patient's symptoms result from stress or from hypovolemic shock?

If you can answer yes to two or more of the following questions, suspect hypovolemic shock and notify the doctor immediately.
• Is the patient's skin cool, clammy, and pale?
• Is he restless, anxious, or confused?
• Is his pulse rapid and thready?
• Is his pulse pressure narrowing?
• Is his urine output low (less than 30 ml/hour)?
• Are his sensory perceptions diminished?
Nursing interventions. Your
Continued

Checking for Hypovolemic Shock
Continued

patient will need emergency intervention to improve ventilation and replace lost fluids. In addition to carefully assessing and monitoring his vital signs, take these other nursing measures during treatment:

• Check for a patent airway and adequate circulation. If pulse and blood pressure are absent, begin CPR.

• Place the patient in a supine position. If he's hemorrhaging severely, elevate his legs 20° to 30°.

• Record blood pressure, pulse rate, peripheral pulses, respiratory rate, and other vital signs every 15 minutes. If systolic blood pressure drops below 80 mm Hg, notify the doctor immediately.

• Monitor the EKG continuously.

• As ordered, start an I.V. with normal saline or lactated Ringer's solution, using a large-bore catheter for easier administration of later blood transfusions. (*Caution:* If your patient in shock has suffered abdominal trauma, in addi-

tion to chest trauma, don't start an I.V. in the leg, since infused fluid may escape through the ruptured vessel into the abdomen.)

• If certified, draw blood for arterial blood gas measurements.

• Administer oxygen by face mask or airway to ensure adequate tissue oxygenation. Adjust the oxygen flow rate according to ABG values.

• The doctor may want to measure the patient's hourly urinary output with a Foley catheter. If output remains below 30 ml/hour, notify the doctor.

• Assess the patient's skin color and temperature frequently. Cold, clammy skin may indicate progressive shock.

• Watch for signs of impending coagulopathy (for example, bruising, petechiae, or bleeding or oozing from the gums or venipuncture site).

• Explain all procedures and provide emotional support to the patient and his family.

Interpreting Test Results

No *single* laboratory test confirms a diagnosis of disseminated intravascular coagulation (DIC). Nevertheless, hematologic lab test results, in conjunction with assessment findings, can strongly support the diagnosis. *Note:* Your hospital may specify a battery of tests, called a *DIC screen*, that includes those blood tests most useful for identifying DIC. Check your lab manual for details.

If drawing blood specimens for blood tests is a nursing responsibility in your hospital, keep the following guidelines in mind.
• Check your hospital's lab manual to determine the correct type and size of collection tube to use for each specimen.
• Draw specimens through your patient's arterial line, if he has one in place. Remember, his condition predisposes him to excessive bleeding from venipuncture sites.
• On the lab slip, note the medications your patient is taking. Many commonly ordered drugs can affect lab values. *Important:* Take special care to clearly note heparin therapy, if your patient is receiving it.
• Note any diseases or conditions your patient has that may affect test results.

Managing DIC: Some Nursing Considerations

In addition to identifying early signs and symptoms, your role in DIC management involves correcting the underlying disorders, compensating for anemia and hypovolemia, and preventing additional bleeding. Follow these guidelines:
• Carefully check your patient's blood study results, especially hemoglobin and hematocrit values and coagulation times.
• Give replacement blood or blood products, as ordered, to replace depleted clotting factors and platelets. Watch for transfusion reactions and fluid overload.
• Assist with mechanical ventilation, peritoneal dialysis, or hemodialysis, as ordered.
• Administer oxygen, as ordered.
• To determine your patient's blood loss, weigh the dressings and linen and record the amount of drainage. *Note:* Don't forget to include blood specimens when you document blood loss.

Continued

SHOCK CARE

Managing DIC: Some Nursing Considerations
Continued

• Weigh the patient at the same time each day in the same or similar clothing, to check his fluid balance, particularly if he has a kidney disorder. In acute DIC, monitor intake and output hourly.

• Watch for bleeding from the gastrointestinal and genitourinary tracts. If you suspect intraabdominal hemorrhage, measure the patient's abdominal girth every 4 hours. Test specimens of gastric secretions, stool, and urine for blood.

• Be alert for signs and symptoms of hypovolemic shock.

• Check I.V. sites frequently for bleeding.

• Limit intramuscular and subcutaneous injections. Apply pressure to injection site for at least 10 minutes to control the bleeding.

• To prevent blood clots from dislodging and causing fresh bleeding, don't scrub bleeding areas.

• Use pressure, cold compresses, and topical hemostatic agents, such as an absorbable gelatin sponge (Gelfoam), to control the bleeding.

• If ordered, give your patient heparin. *Note:* Heparin therapy to treat DIC is controversial, because heparin disrupts the clotting cascade. Heparin is contraindicated if the patient has brain damage or dysfunction, or if he has a necrotizing lesion.

• If ordered, give your patient aminocaproic acid (Amicar*), an antifibrinolytic agent. Because this drug may cause clots in vital organs, giving it is also controversial.

• Protect your patient from injury. Turn and position him carefully. Enforce bed rest during bleeding episodes and pad the bed's side rails if your patient is agitated.

• Tell co-workers of the patient's tendency to hemorrhage.

• Provide gentle mouth care. Remember, your patient's gums may bleed easily.

• Avoid using adhesive tape. The force needed to remove it may damage skin, causing bleeding.

• To help control pain from tissue ischemia, administer analgesics that don't contain aspirin, as ordered.

• Perform passive range-of-motion exercises on your patient during nonbleeding periods to reduce joint and muscle pain. Avoid giving back rubs or skin massages because these may promote bleeding.

• Because DIC may cause hemorrhaging in major organs, watch your patient for signs and symptoms of cerebral, gastrointestinal, and hepatic hemorrage.

• Provide emotional support for the patient and his family.

• Document all patient care.

*Available in the United States and Canada

Do's and Don'ts for Using MAST Effectively

MAST (Medical Anti-Shock Trousers) counteracts bleeding and hypovolemia by slowing or stopping arterial bleeding; by forcing any available blood from the lower body to the heart, brain, and any other vital organ in the upper body; and by preventing return of the available circulating blood volume to the lower extremities.

Do's:
● While patient is wearing MAST: monitor vital signs, blood pressure, apical and radial pulse rate, and respirations; check extremities for pedal pulses, color, warmth, and numbness; and make sure MAST is not too constricting.

● Take MAST off only when: A doctor is present; fluids are available for transfusion; and anesthesia and surgical teams are ready for the patient.
● To clean: Wash with warm soap and water; or air dry and store.

Don'ts:
● Don't apply MAST if: Positions of wounds show or suggest intrathoracic or intracranial major vascular injury; patient has open-extremity bleeding, pulmonary edema, or trauma above the level of MAST application.
● When cleaning, don't autoclave or clean with solvents.

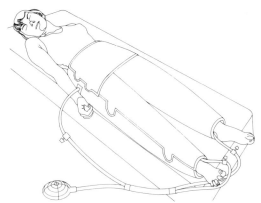

Comparing I.V. Replacement Fluids

No matter what triggered your patient's hypovolemic shock, restoring circulating fluid volume is the key to treatment. Use this chart to review the basics about commonly ordered I.V. replacement fluids.

Note: If your patient has lost a large volume of blood, he'll also need a blood transfusion.

LACTATED RINGER'S INJECTION (HARTMANN'S SOLUTION)

Electrolyte solution consisting of sodium chloride, potassium chloride, calcium chloride, and sodium lactate in water
Indications
For initial fluid replacement in all types of hypovolemia. If blood loss is less than 1,500 ml, lactated Ringer's injection may be the only fluid necessary.
Advantages
• Closely resembles blood plasma; may be used as an emergency volume expander while blood is being typed and cross matched
• Contains electrolyte content needed for adequate kidney function
• Rarely causes adverse reactions
• Is inexpensive and readily available
Disadvantage
None significant
Nursing considerations
• Use cautiously if the patient has renal failure or dysfunction, congestive heart failure, hypoprotein-

emia, or pulmonary edema.
• Monitor patient closely for signs of fluid overload.

0.9% SODIUM CHLORIDE (NORMAL SALINE SOLUTION)

Isotonic noncolloidal electrolyte solution
Indications
To treat dehydration or sodium depletion
Advantages
• May be used as an emergency plasma expander while whole blood is being typed and cross matched
• Is inexpensive and readily available
Disadvantage
• May cause these side effects: hypernatremia, hypokalemia, and hyperchloremic metabolic acidosis
Nursing considerations
• Use cautiously if the patient has congestive heart failure, renal dysfunction, or hypoproteinemia.
• Monitor the patient constantly for signs of pulmonary edema and fluid overload.
• Monitor the patient's serum electrolytes closely.

Continued

Comparing I.V. Replacement Fluids
Continued

DEXTROSE 5% IN WATER

Hypotonic noncolloidal solution
Indications
To maintain water balance and supply calories necessary for cell metabolism
Advantage
• Is inexpensive and readily available
Disadvantage
• Causes red blood cell clumping, so can't be given with blood
Nursing considerations
• Dextrose in water is not a solution of choice for shock (unless shock is caused entirely by water deprivation). Use it only to establish an emergency I.V. line. As soon as possible, switch to lactated Ringer's injection, as ordered.
• Maintain accurate fluid intake and output records.

DEXTRAN

Synthetic colloidal solution that simulates albumin's effects; usually given with 0.9% sodium chloride solution (normal saline solution); available in both high molecular and low molecular weights
Indications
As a plasma expander in shock caused by excessive plasma loss

Advantage
• Provides plasma volume expansion and early fluid replacement when compatible blood or blood products aren't available
Disadvantages
• May interfere with blood typing and cross matching because it coats the cells
• May cause these side effects: allergic reaction (for example, anaphylactoid reaction), decreased hemoglobin and hematocrit levels, and kidney failure
Nursing considerations
• Use cautiously when shock is caused by hemorrhage, because dextran increases the tendency of blood to ooze from wounds (usually without demonstrable coagulation changes, however).
• Draw blood specimens for typing and cross matching *before* beginning the infusion.
• Don't administer as a whole blood substitute.
• Don't use *high* molecular weight dextrans (for example, Dextran 75*) interchangeably with *low* molecular weight dextrans (for example, Dextran 40). They differ significantly.
• Give no more than 1 liter/day, as ordered.

Continued

*Available in the United States and Canada

SHOCK CARE

Comparing I.V. Replacement Fluids
Continued

HETASTARCH (HES)

Synthetic colloidal solution
Indications
As a plasma expander
Advantages
• Compared with albumin and 0.9% sodium chloride solutions, HES significantly raises colloid osmotic pressure. Since more fluid stays in the vessels, the patient may need less fluid volume replacement. Also, he's at low risk of pulmonary edema.
• Unlike albumin solutions, has no apparent effect on renal function

• Is unlikely to cause an allergic reaction
• May provide adequate fluid volume replacement for patients who refuse blood transfusions for religious reasons
• Has a long shelf life and is inexpensive
Disadvantage
None significant
Nursing considerations
• Use cautiously if the patient has a severe bleeding disorder, severe heart failure, or renal failure.
• Look for signs of fluid overload.
   Note: HES affects prothrombin time (PT) and plasma thrombin time (PTT).

Nursing Tip

Quick check for I.V.s: When you have several patients receiving I.V. fluids, a quick way to check on the absorption rate is to attach a piece of adhesive tape lengthwise to each bottle. At the top of the tape, mark the time the solution was hung. At the bottom of the tape, mark the time the solution should be aborsbed. Midway between these two labels, mark the time when half the amount of the solution should be absorbed. With these markings, you'll be able to see at a glance whether the solutions are being absorbed on schedule.
—SYLVIA E. PLATT, RN

Using a blood pressure cuff to locate veins: If you have to insert an I.V. in the dorsum of a patient's hand and can't find his veins, simplify the search. Apply a blood pressure cuff to the patient's arm below the elbow. Then pump the cuff to 40 mm Hg and wait about 2 minutes for the small veins to appear on the hand.
   The blood pressure cuff helps you locate veins better than a conventional tourniquet.
—LARRY K. KING, RN

SHOCK CARE

Combating Burn Shock: Your Role

To prevent or treat burn shock, your first priority is fluid replacement. How much fluid does your patient need? When dealing with burn shock, you needn't wrestle with cumbersome formulas for the answer. In simple terms, your patient needs whatever amount of fluid is necessary to maintain his urine output at more than 50 ml/hour. Later, when the threat of burn shock is past, the doctor will adjust the I.V. fluid flow rate according to the patient's condition.

The I.V. solution you'll administer depends on the hospital's policy and the doctor's preference. He may order lactated Ringer's solution, adding 25 g of albumin per liter after 24 hours. If the patient suffers from metabolic acidosis, you may give sodium bicarbonate, too.

Your role in reversing burn shock is critical. Follow these guidelines:
• Rapidly assess the severity of your patient's burns, using either the Berkow method or the Rule of Nines (see page 130).
• Insert a large-bore I.V. catheter, or prepare to assist the doctor in doing so. If an unburned site is unavailable, he'll probably insert the catheter through burned tissue, to avoid venous cutdown. (Venous cutdown further compromises damaged veins.)

• Obtain venous blood specimens, as ordered, for laboratory studies and blood cross matching.
• Obtain arterial blood specimens, as ordered, to determine blood pH and arterial blood gas values.
• Insert an indwelling (Foley) catheter.
• Begin fluid replacement therapy, as ordered, and closely monitor urine output. Expect to administer fluid as rapidly as possible, until urine output resumes. Then adjust the flow rate, as ordered, to maintain urine output at more than 50 ml/hour.
• Regularly (at least hourly) document the patient's urine output, urine specific gravity, blood pressure, pulse rate and rhythm, respiratory rate, and level of consciousness. Also, note whether the patient is having difficulty breathing.
• Readjust the I.V. flow rate, as ordered. When the patient's urine output is above 50 ml/hour for 2 consecutive hours (or according to hospital policy), the doctor may begin reducing the I.V. flow rate by 50 ml/hour.

Important: The threat of burn shock usually ends within 48 hours of injury. If the patient isn't responding to fluid replacement therapy in this time, suspect an underlying problem, such as respiratory, cardiac, or renal failure.

SHOCK CARE

Using the Rule of Nines

For an adult patient, the Rule of Nines provides a quick, reliable guide to burn severity. As you probably know, this assessment method divides the body surface area (BSA) into areas representing 9%, or multiples of 9%, as shown here. To use this technique, match the areas where your patient is burned to the corresponding areas on the diagram. Then total the percentages to get a rough estimate of burn severity.

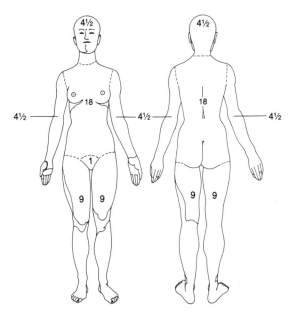

Guidelines for Fluid Replacement

While fluids are being replaced, assess your patient's response and use it to titrate the rate of fluid replacement. But use caution in giving massive fluid replacement to elderly and pediatric patients and to anyone with a history of heart failure. Osmotic diuretics or low-dose dopamine infusions may be necessary to maintain adequate urine output and prevent fluid overload in these patients or to aid myoglobin clearance in patients with deep-muscle damage.

ASSESSMENT FACTORS	NURSING CONSIDERATIONS
Intake and output (hourly)	Maintain minimum urine output at 30 to 50 ml/hr in an adult, 0.5 to 1 ml/kg/hr in a child, or 70 to 100 ml/hr in a patient with a deep burn injury affecting muscle tissue, to prevent renal failure from myoglobinuria.
Vital signs (every 15 minutes to hourly)	Maintain the patient's blood pressure above 90/60. Increase the fluid infusion rate and notify the doctor if the patient's blood pressure drops more than 20 mm Hg below baseline or if his pulse rises above 110 beats/minute.
Mental status (continuously)	Note changes such as restlessness, confusion, or agitation in a previously quiet patient, indicating poor cerebral perfusion.
Body weight (same time daily)	Expect the patient to gain weight during the first 48 to 72 hours, due to third-space fluid shifting. Thereafter, expect the patient's weight to slowly decrease toward normal dry weight.

Continued

SHOCK CARE

Guidelines for Fluid Replacement
Continued

ASSESSMENT FACTORS	NURSING CONSIDERATIONS
Respiratory status (hourly)	Check the patient's breath sounds for rales, and note dyspnea, which may indicate fluid overload. If rales or dyspnea is present, decrease the fluid administration rate and notify the doctor.
Cardiac status (frequently)	Monitor the EKG continuously with an elderly patient or a patient with a history of heart failure, and auscultate heart sounds at least hourly; notify the doctor if rales, dysrhythmias, or abnormal heart sounds—which may indicate fluid overload—develop.
Blood tests (at least daily) • hematocrit • sodium	Notify the doctor if the patient's values are elevated (possibly indicating underhydration) or decreased (possibly indicating overhydration). He may change the infusion rate and the type of fluid administered and may order a blood transfusion. (*Note:* Expect an initial rise in hematocrit values.)
Urine specific gravity (every 4 hours)	If elevated, expect to increase the infusion rate; or if decreased, to decrease the infusion rate.

SHOCK CARE

Fluid Replacement for Burn Patients

FORMULA	ELECTROLYTE CONTAINING SOLUTION	COLLOIDS	DEXTROSE
	FIRST 24 HOURS POSTBURN		
Baxter (Parkland)	Ringer's lactate—4 ml/ kg/% burn	Not used	Not used
Hypertonic sodium solution	Volume of fluid containing 250 mEq of sodium per liter to maintain hourly urinary output of 30 mg/ml	Not used	Not used
Modified Brooke	Ringer's lactate—2 ml/ kg/% burn	Not used	Not used
Burn budget of F.D. Moore	Ringer's lactate— 1,000 to 4,000 ml; 0.5 normal saline—1,200 ml	7.5% of body weight	1,500 to 5,000 ml
Evans	Normal saline— 1 ml/kg/% burn	1 ml/kg/% burn	2,000 ml
Brooke	Ringer's lactate— 1.5 ml/kg/% burn	0.5 ml/kg/% burn	2,000 ml

Continued

Fluid Replacement for Burn Patients
Continued

FORMULA	ELECTROLYTE CONTAINING SOLUTION	COLLOIDS	DEXTROSE
	SECOND 24 HOURS POSTBURN		
Burn budget of F.D. Moore	Ringer's lactate— 1,000 to 4,000 ml; 0.5 normal saline—1,200 ml	2.5% of body weight	1,500 to 5,000 ml
Evans	½ of first 24-hour requirement	½ of first 24-hour requirement	2,000 ml
Brooke	½ to ¾ of first 24-hour requirement	½ to ¾ of first 24-hour requirement	2,000 ml
Parkland	Not used	20% to 60% of calculated plasma volume (within 24 to 32 hours)	As necessary to maintain urinary output
Hypertonic sodium solution	⅓ isotonic salt solution orally, up to 3,500-ml limit	Not used	Not used
Modified Brooke	Not used	0.3 to 0.5 ml/kg/% burn	As necessary to maintain urinary output

Classic Symptoms Late

Expect shock in any condition where it's a likely complication: in anaphylaxis; anoxia; any condition associated with fluid loss or sequestered fluid; heart failure from any cause; major blood flow obstruction; any severe infection; and endocrine and metabolic disorders. Be ready to start treatment at the first signs of shock. *Watch for these warning signs:*

• *Skin changes* (temperature and color) reflect tissue oxygenation and perfusion. Continuing cold, clammy skin during fluid replacement signals continuing peripheral vascular constriction. Flushing and sweating indicate overheating. Continuing pallor and cyanosis in a shock patient generally indicate tissue hypoxia.

• *Blood pressure and pulse:* Rapid pulse may be the first sign of shock, whereas a drop in blood pressure is often a *late* sign.

Eventually systolic pressure drops 30 mm Hg or more.

• *Respiration* becomes rapid and shallow. Such air hunger is a common early sign of shock as the body tries to compensate for tissue hypoxia. Slow breathing—2 to 3 breaths per minute—appears late in shock after failure of the compensatory mechanisms.

• *Temperature* usually drops below normal with hemorrhagic shock. Again, watch for change: Gradually rising temperature may signal developing sepsis.

• *Restlessness* is common in early shock and indicates hypoxia.

• *Urine output* below 30 ml per hour signals marked reduction in renal blood flow—a sign of severe shock. When you see decreasing urine output and hypovolemia, increase fluid infusion rate to the maximum and call a doctor.

Classification of Shock

If you classify shock in two different groups — cardiogenic or central, and peripheral — you may understand its dynamics more easily. Cardiogenic shock refers to those cases resulting from dysfunction of the heart itself. An impairment in cardiac emptying or filling can lead to shock.

Peripheral shock includes those cases of hypovolemia or of capillary blood pooling, as in patients with hemorrhage or septicemia.

Remember — more than one condition may precipitate shock. Others may aggravate the situation, creating a vicious circle. Your understanding of shock and all its facets is vital to patient care.

Classification of Shock

DEFINITION	PHYSIOLOGICAL DISTURBANCE	ETIOLOGY
Peripheral Decreased blood volume, hypovolemia	*Hemogenic* (loss of blood)	hemorrhage
	Traumatic (loss of plasma)	burns or trauma
	Dehydration	loss of fluids via kidneys gastrointestinal tract sweat glands
Pooling of blood	*Endotoxic* (septic)	bacterial or viral infection
	Anaphylactic	histamine or histamine-like substance
	Neurogenic (reflex or neurohumoral)	pain drugs (anesthesia, soporifics), heat stroke
Cardiogenic (central) Primary insufficiency of cardiac output due to impaired pumping action	*Myocardial*	myocardial infarction, acute myocarditis, terminal failure
	Valvular	rupture of valve cusp
Secondary insufficiency due to filling defect	*Mechanical*	pulmonary embolism, pericardial tamponade, valvular obstruction by atrial tumor, or thrombus
	Functional	ectopic-tachycardias, severe dysrhythmias

Therapy Based on Peripheral Resistance Changes

PERIPHERAL RESISTANCE	THERAPY
Increased	Correct the causative condition with vasoconstrictors, digitalis, corticosteroids, fluids, vasodilators, isoproterenol, oxygen
Increased	Blood, plasma, dextran, corticosteroids, vasoconstrictors, oxygen
Increased	Plasma, isotonic, hypotonic, or hypertonic solutions, vasoconstrictors
Increased	Corticosteroids, fluids, antiobiotics, vasoconstrictors
Decreased	Epinephrine, antihistamines
Decreased	Vasoconstrictors

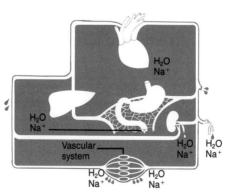

What Causes Cardiogenic Shock?

Although left ventricular failure from myocardial infarction is the most common cause of cardiogenic shock, it's not the *only* cause. Other possible causes fall into the categories that are listed here:

Chronic progressive heart diseases, causing heart cell degeneration with reduced contractility. Examples include congestive cardiomyopathies, myocarditis, and atherosclerotic heart disease.

Injury or disease, causing mechanical failure. Examples include papillary muscle rupture, interventricular septum rupture, ventricular wall rupture with acute tamponade, severe valvular disease, atrial myxoma (a benign tumor), mural thrombus (heart-chamber wall thrombus), and ventricular aneurysm that collects blood and lessens the heart's contractility.

Obstruction of venous return, reducing preload. Examples include tension pneumothorax and cardiac tamponade.

Dysrhythmias, especially combined with another condition.

Taking the First Steps

Do you suspect that your patient is going into cardiogenic shock? Take these steps:
• Call the doctor immediately.
• Administer oxygen.
• Start an I.V. or check the patency of the existing I.V. line.
• Insert an indwelling (Foley) catheter, and measure urine output frequently.
• Draw blood specimens for arterial blood gas measurements and cardiac isoenzyme studies, as ordered.
• Obtain a 12-lead EKG.
• As ordered, administer I.V. drugs, such as dopamine hydrochloride, norepinephrine, or nitroprusside sodium.
• Place your patient in low Fowler position. However, if he's unconscious or semiconscious, place him in a supine position to encourage maximum blood flow to the brain.
• Assist with tracheal intubation, if indicated.
• Prepare your patient for transfer to the cardiac care unit (CCU).
• Provide emotional support to your patient and his family. In easy-to-understand terms, explain all procedures as well as what to expect after the patient's transfer to the CCU.

Neurogenic and Hypovolemic Shock: Identifying the Differences

Do you know how to differentiate signs and symptoms of neurogenic shock from those of hypovolemic shock? If not, you should. Remember that inappropriate nursing actions taken as a result of confusing these shock types may be fatal to your patient.

Suppose, for example, you incorrectly identify decreased blood volume as the cause of your patient's shock, and increase the I.V. flow rate. This could be dangerous if your patient is really suffering from neurogenic shock. Why? Because fluid volume overload may occur when vasomotor tone is restored, for example, by vasopressor drugs. If your patient has a preexisting heart condition, volume overload could lead to congestive heart failure or pulmonary edema—both potentially fatal complications. So, although your patient may need fluid replacement to restore circulating volume, you must give fluids with caution.

As you can see, your ability to differentiate between these shock types is crucial. To refresh your memory of the signs and symptoms of each, study this chart.

HYPOVOLEMIC SHOCK

- Cold, clammy, pale skin
- Low blood pressure
- Increased pulse rate
- Decreased temperature
- Increased respiratory rate
- Blood or fluid loss exceeding 20% of total circulatory volume.

NEUROGENIC SHOCK

- Warm, dry, possibly flushed skin
- Normal blood pressure (which may fail quickly) or low blood pressure
- Full, regular pulse
- Profound bradycardia (possibly)
- Poikilothermy (body temperature varies with environmental temperature)
- Increased respiratory rate (possibly)
- No blood or fluid loss
- Full neck veins (possibly)
- History of predisposing condition (for example, deep general or spinal anesthesia; head or spinal cord trauma).

SHOCK CARE

What Happens in Neurogenic Shock

In neurogenic shock, the major problem is altered blood vessel capacity. A neurologic insult disrupts sympathetic nerve impulse transmission from the brain's vasomotor center, causing unopposed parasympathetic stimulation. This causes vasomotor tone loss, resulting in massive vasodilation: the vascular bed increases in size and blood capacity. So, even though the patient's blood volume isn't actually depleted, it's still inadequate to fill the enlarged vascular bed. The result? Relative hypovolemia, decreased venous return, and decreased cardiac output, which trigger the body's compensatory mechanisms. Usually, these mechanisms are successful—vasoconstriction occurs, reducing the relative hypovolemia and improving vasomotor tone—or the condition spontaneously resolves itself.

Depending on your patient's condition, and on the doctor's order, to identify neurogenic shock you may perform a neurocheck every 15 minutes or once every 2 hours. Do neurochecks frequently in these instances:
• before and after a procedure for which a spinal anesthetic was used
• before and after a procedure requiring deep general anesthesia
• after head or spinal cord trauma
• whenever your patient's level of consciousness, motor and sensory response, or pupillary response changes significantly.

What's Your Role?

To prevent complications while a patient is in neurogenic shock, follow these guidelines:
• Place your patient in a supine position on a bed or stretcher. But if you suspect cerebral edema, reposition him in a 20° to 30° Fowler position, if ordered. Never place a neurogenic shock patient in Trendelenburg position. If ordered, however, you may elevate his legs to encourage venous return.
• Monitor your patient's vital signs, as well as fluid intake and output. Perform frequent neurochecks. Watch for changes and report significant ones.
• Start an I.V., if ordered, to provide a route for drugs and fluid.
• Insert an indwelling (Foley) catheter, if ordered, to prevent fluid retention and to monitor his urine output.
• If necessary, insert a nasogastric tube, as ordered, to reduce gastric distention from ileus and reduce the risk of vomiting.
• Administer drugs, as ordered.
• Reassure your patient.
• Document everything.

SHOCK CARE

Comparing Hypovolemic to Warm Septic Shock

HYPOVOLEMIC SHOCK
Skin: Cool, clammy, pale
Blood pressure: Below normal
Pulse pressure: Narrowing
Pulse quality: Weak, thready
Urine output: Below normal (less than 30 ml/hour)

WARM SEPTIC SHOCK
Skin: Warm, dry, flushed
Blood pressure: Normal or slightly above normal
Pulse pressure: Widening
Pulse quality: Full and possibly bounding
Urine output: Normal or possibly above normal

Recognizing Toxic Shock Syndrome

Toxic shock syndrome (TSS) is an acute form of septic shock caused by infection with *Staphylococcus aureus*—a gram-positive bacterium that may invade any part of your patient's body. Once *S. aureus* has invaded every part of your patient's body, the bacteria secrete enterotoxins that cause TSS.

TSS is most common in menstruating women using tampons, but it strikes patients of either sex and any age. On the average, two new cases are reported each day in the United States, and two deaths occur each month.

TSS is difficult to recognize and diagnose. No positive diagnostic tests exist, the onset of TSS is insidious, and its systemic signs and symptoms mimic many other diseases, including viral influenza, food poisoning, scarlet fever, Kawasaki disease, and Rocky Mountain spotted fever.

Remember to consider the possibility of TSS whenever you see a patient with this clinical picture:
• fever above 102° F. (38.9° C.)
• systolic blood pressure below 90 mm Hg
• diffuse rash
• signs and symptoms indicating involvement of at least three body areas (mucous membranes or GI, musculoskeletal, renal, hepatic, hematologic, or central nervous systems)
• negative blood and cerebrospinal fluid culture tests; negative serologic tests for measles, leptospirosis, and Rocky Mountain spotted fever
• positive results of testing for *S. aureus* cultured from the nose, throat, vagina, or any wound
• squamation (especially of the palms and soles) a week or more after the onset of signs and symptoms.

What Happens in Septic Shock

Massive infection, most commonly from gram-negative bacteria, is the cause of septic shock. As the body fights the infection, the bacteria die, releasing endotoxins. These endotoxins, through as-yet-unknown mechanisms, impair cell metabolism and damage surrounding tissues. The damaged cells release lysosomal enzymes and histamine. The lysosomal enzymes travel through the bloodstream to other tissues, causing more cell damage. They also trigger the release of bradykinin, a powerful vasoactive substance. Combined with histamine from the damaged cells, bradykinin causes massive peripheral vasodilation and increased capillary permeability (the so-called warm stage of septic shock). This leads to increased third-space fluid shifting and relative hypovolemia. The heart's preload, afterload, and stoke volume all decrease, triggering compensation (the cool stage) in an attempt to stave off decompensation (the cold stage) and death.

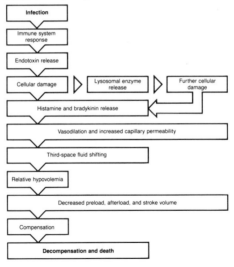

Calculating Flow Rates

To calculate the right flow rate for your patient, answer these questions:
• How much solution did the doctor order?
• How much time is allowed for delivery?

Take the amount of solution to be administerd and divide it by the delivery time; for example,

$$\frac{1000 \text{ ml}}{8 \text{ hours}} = 125 \text{ ml per hour.}$$

Now, decide which type of drip system you're using. If you're delivering a lot of fluid in a short time, use a macrodrip system. The macrodrip, depending on the manufacturer, takes 10, 15, or 20 drops to deliver 1 ml. If you're delivering a small amount of fluid over a long time, use a microdrip system. The microdrip takes 60 drops to deliver 1 ml.

Insert your answers into this formula:

$$\frac{\text{drops per ml}}{60 \text{ minutes per hour}}$$

$$\frac{\times \text{ amount of fluid per hour}}{1}$$

= drops per minute

If you're using a macrodrip system, your equation will look like one of these:

$^{10}/_{60} \times {}^{125}/_{1} = {}^{125}/_{6} = 21$ drops per minute;

$^{15}/_{60} \times {}^{125}/_{1} = {}^{125}/_{4} = 31$ drops per minute;

$^{20}/_{60} \times {}^{125}/_{1} = {}^{125}/_{3} = 41$ drops per minute.

If you're using a microdrip system, your equation will look like this:

$^{60}/_{60} \times {}^{125}/_{1} = 125$ drops per minute.

After you've determined the rate, setting the flow is easy. When you've established your I.V. line, slowly open the clamp to start fluid dripping into the drip chamber. Hold your watch close to the chamber, and time the drips for 1 minute. Open or close the clamp, as needed, to adjust the drip rate. *Remember:* Anytime the clamp slips, for whatever reason, or the patient makes a sudden move, the drip rate may be affected. Check it periodically, using the method described above. Remind the patient and his family not to tamper with the clamp.

I.V. Admixtures: Preventing Incompatibility and Instability

An incompatibility is an undesired physiochemical reaction between a drug and a primary container, a primary solution, or another drug. The action destroys the drug's therapeutic effect or creates new and unwanted ones. You can prevent this type of reaction by knowing about the drugs and solutions you're mixing.

Stability refers to how long a drug retains, within specified limits, the same properties and characteristics it possessed when manufactured. The limit on stability for all drugs has been set at 10% by the United States government. So when a drug is said to be stable, at least 90% of its properties are effective until a specific date. If it loses more than 10% of its effectiveness, it's considered unstable. The general term incompatibility, in practical usage, refers to instability as well.

Types of incompatibilities

● Physical: Most physical incompatibilities result from inadequate solubility and from acid/base reactions. A physical incompatibility has occurred when you see precipitation, color change, gas release, or cloudiness in the bottle. For example, when diazepam is mixed with 5% dextrose in water, the solution becomes cloudy.

● Chemical: A chemical incompatibility, which may not always be visible, is the irreversible breakdown of a drug, producing therapeutically inactive or toxic products. For example, mixing carbenicillin disodiumicinsulate deactivates the gentamicin. Some chemical instability can't be prevented. Take, for example, hydrolysis and oxidation.

Hydrolysis most commonly occurs in hyperalimentation solutions and fat emulsions. This reaction produces substances that may be more acidic than the original drug, may discolor the solution, and may be toxic or sensitizing. Hydrolysis doesn't necessarily alter the drug's therapeutic effect.

Continued

OTHER
CRITICAL CARE CONCERNS

I.V. Admixtures: Preventing Incompatibility and Instability

Continued

Oxidation occurs when the drug or solution experiences electron or hydrogen loss, or an oxygen increase. It causes the drug or solution to turn pink, red, or brown and makes it therapeutically ineffective.

Four factors affect compatibility

• Concentration of the drug—the stronger the drug's concentration, the swifter it may become incompatible or unstable.

• Length of contact time—the longer the drugs are in contact (either because they're prepared before they're needed or because of long administration time), the greater the chance that the mixture will become incompatible or unstable.

• Ionic strength of the drug—the less the drug's ionic strength, the greater the chance of incompatibility or instability.

• pH level of the mixture—when a drug's added to a primary solution, the solution's pH may be altered considerably. Many drugs, especially antibiotics, are unstable in alkaline (pH above 8) or in acidic (pH below 4) solutions. Some solutions, such as fructose, decompose if they're made alkaline by the addition of a drug like calcium, which causes the pH to exceed 7. This admixture is considered incompatible.

What buffers do

Buffers are substances added to drugs or solutions during manufacture to maintain a desired pH. Although drugs often have their own buffer, it's usually too weak to counteract the pH change that occurs when the drug's added to a strongly acidic or alkaline I.V. solution. This change in pH can cause the drug to separate from the primary solution. Potassium penicillin G, for example, is considered most stable in the pH range of 6 to 7. But if you add it to a dextrose 5% in water solution, along with other

Continued

I.V. Admixtures: Preventing Incompatibility and Instability
Continued

highly buffered drugs that make the solution alkaline (amphotericin B or cephalothin solution), potassium penicillin G rapidly deteriorates. The ideal pH for I.V. fluids is approximately 7.4, the pH of blood.

General precautions when preparing I.V. admixtures

• Add one drug at a time to the primary I.V. solution. Mix and examine it thoroughly before adding the next drug.

• Add the most concentrated or most soluble drug to the solution first, since some incompatibilities, such as precipitates, require a certain concentration or amount of time to develop. Mix it well, and then add the dilute drugs.

• Remember that chemical analogues or families of drugs react similarly, though not necessarily identically. If one drug in a class is incompatible with the desired solution, other drugs in that class may be incompatible too.

• You'll find some precipitates are too fine or too clear to detect visually. Using colored additives may make it even harder. You should add additives such as riboflavin in vitamin B complex (yellow color) to the solution last to avoid masking possible precipitates or cloudiness.

• Even though contact time has been shortened with the use of minicontainers and backcheck valves, you must always check for compatibility and stability.

• If you don't have a clear understanding of the compatibility or stability you're using, check the manufacturer's recommendations, and consult with a pharmacist.

• Because of the complexity of this subject, many hospitals allow only registered pharmacists to prepare admixtures. But if this isn't your hospital's policy, make sure, before you begin, to have several drug references handy.

OTHER
CRITICAL CARE CONCERNS

Complications from I.V. Therapy

INFILTRATION

Possible causes
• Needle or catheter displacement (either partial or complete)
• Leakage of blood around needle or catheter (especially likely in an older patient whose tissues have lost their elasticity)

Signs and symptoms
• Coolness of skin around site
• Swelling around site, which may or may not be painful
• Swelling of entire limb
• Absence of blood backflow. If a tourniquet's applied above the site, the infusion continues to run.
• Sluggish flow rate

Nursing considerations
• Discontinue the infusion, and remove the needle or catheter immediately.
• If the infiltration's caught within a half hour and the swelling's small, apply ice. Otherwise, apply warm, wet compresses to encourage absorption.
• Restart I.V. in another limb.
• Document what you've done.

Prevention tips
• Use a splint to stabilize the needle or catheter when the site's over a joint or the patient's active.
• Palpate occasionally to confirm proper needle position. When a needle's placed correctly in a superficial vein, you can usually feel it easily.

THROMBOPHLEBITIS

Possible causes
• Injury to the vein, either during venipuncture or from needle movement later
• Irritation to the vein caused by the following: long-term therapy, irritating or incompatible additives, or use of a vein that's too small to handle the amount or type of solution
• Sluggish flow rate, which allows a clot to form at the end of the needle or catheter

Signs and symptoms
• Sluggish flow rate
• Edema in limb
• A vein that's sore, hard, cordlike, and warm to the touch. It may look like a red line above the venipuncture site.

Nursing considerations
• Discontinue the infusion and remove the needle or catheter immediately.
• Apply warm, wet compresses.
• Notify doctor.
• Restart I.V. in another limb.
• Document what you've done.
• *Important:* In the case of a sluggish flow rate, never try to irrigate the line. In addition to increasing the risk of infection, you may flush a clot into the bloodstream, causing an embolus.

Continued

OTHER
CRITICAL CARE CONCERNS

Complications from I.V. Therapy
Continued

THROMBOPHLEBITIS
Continued

Prevention tips
• If you have to use an irritating additive, try to find a vein large enough to dilute it. Dilute irritating additives with diluents, if possible.
• Make sure drug additives are compatible.
• Keep the infusion flowing at the prescribed rate.
• Stabilize the needle or catheter with a splint, if necessary.

CIRCULATORY OVERLOAD

Possible causes
• Too much fluid
• Fluid delivered too fast
Signs and symptoms
• Rise in blood pressure and central venous pressure (CVP)
• Dilation of veins, with neck veins sometimes visibly engorged
• Rapid breathing, shortness of breath, rales
• Wide variance between liquid input and urine output
Nursing considerations
• Slow the infusion to a keep-vein-open (KVO) rate.
• Raise patient's head.
• Keep him warm.
• Monitor vital signs.
• Administer oxygen, if permitted.
• Notify doctor.
• Document what you've done.

Prevention tips
• Be aware of the patient's cardiovascular status and history.
• Tell the doctor if the fluid volume or flow rate may be more than the patient can tolerate.
• Monitor the patient's urine output.

AIR EMBOLISM

(Air embolisms pose a greater risk and are more common with central lines than with peripheral ones.)
Possible causes
• Container allowed to run dry
• Air in tubing
• Loose connections
Signs and symptoms
• Blood pressure drop
• Rise in CVP
• Weak, rapid pulse
• Cyanosis
• Loss of consciousness
Nursing considerations
• Turn the patient on his left side, and lower the head of the bed. If air's entered his heart chambers, this position may keep it on the right side of the heart. The pulmonary artery will then absorb small air bubbles.
• Check system for leaks.
• Give oxygen if allowed.
• Notify doctor immediately.
• Document what you've done.

Continued

Complications from I.V. Therapy
Continued

AIR EMBOLISM
Continued

Prevention tips
• Clear all air from the tubing before attaching it to the patient.
• Change containers before they're empty.
• Make sure all connections are secure.

CATHETER EMBOLISM

(Catheter embolisms are more common with inside-the-needle catheters [INC] than with outside-the-needle catheters [ONC].)

Possible causes
• Withdrawing the catheter before the needle or attempting to rethread a catheter with a needle
• Failure to secure the catheter to the skin adequately

Signs and symptoms
• Discomfort along the vein in which the catheter fragment's lodged
• Blood pressure drop
• Rise in CVP
• Weak, rapid pulse
• Cyanosis
• Loss of consciousness

Nursing considerations
• Discontinue I.V.
• Apply tourniquet above site. You may be able to stop the catheter from migrating farther.

• Have patient X-rayed to confirm embolism.
• Document what you've done.

Prevention tips
• Remember to withdraw needle and catheter together after an unsuccessful venipuncture attempt.
• Take special care when taping or withdrawing an INC.

INFECTION OF VENIPUNCTURE SITE

Possible cause
• Poor aseptic techniques; for example, failure to keep the site clean or to change I.V. equipment regularly

Signs and symptoms
• Swelling and soreness at site
• Foul-smelling discharge

Nursing considerations
• Discontinue infusion, and remove needle or catheter immediately. Send I.V. equipment to the lab for bacterial analysis.
• Culture drainage.
• Clean site, apply antimicrobial ointment, and cover with sterile gauze pad.
• Restart I.V. in another limb.
• Document what you've done.

Prevention tips
• Review and improve aseptic technique.
• *Remember:* Wash your hands thoroughly before beginning any I.V. procedure.

Continued

OTHER
CRITICAL CARE CONCERNS

Complications from I.V. Therapy
Continued

ALLERGIC REACTION

Possible cause
• Sensitivity to an I.V. fluid (especially an additive)
Signs and symptoms
• Itching
• Rash
• Shortness of breath
Nursing considerations
• Slow infusion to KVO rate.
• Notify doctor.
• Document what you've done.
Prevention tips
• Ask the patient if he has any allergies before beginning venipuncture procedures. Remember, he may have a sensitivity to iodine used as a skin prep.

SYSTEMIC INFECTION

(more common with plastic catheters than with metal needles)
Possible causes
• Poor aseptic technique
• Contamination of equipment during manufacture, storage, or use
• Irrigation of clogged I.V.
Signs and symptoms
• Sudden rise in temperature and pulse
• Chills and shaking
• Blood pressure changes
Nursing considerations
• Look for other sources of infection first. Culture urine, sputum, and blood, as ordered.

• Discontinue the I.V. immediately, and send all equipment to the lab for bacterial analysis.
• Restart I.V. in another limb.
• Notify doctor.
• Document what you've done.
Prevention tips
• Take care not to contaminate the site when bathing the patient.
• If the system's accidentally disconnected, don't rejoin it. Replace parts with sterile equipment.

SPEED SHOCK

Possible causes
• Drugs administered too quickly
• Improper administration of bolus infusions
Signs and symptoms
• Flushed face
• Headache
• Tight feeling in chest
• Irregular pulse
• Loss of consciousness
• Shock
• Cardiac arrest
Nursing considerations
• Discontinue drug infusion.
• Begin an infusion of dextrose 5% in water at KVO rate. You must keep the vein open for emergency treatment.
• Notify doctor immediately.
• Document what you've done.
Prevention tips
• Keep infusion flowing at prescribed rate.

Detecting Complications of Intravenous Hyperalimentation (IVH)

HYPERGLYCEMIA

Causes
Overly rapid IVH delivery rate, lowered glucose tolerance, excessive total dextrose load

Signs and symptoms
Glycosuria, nausea, vomiting, diarrhea, confusion, headache, and lethargy. Untreated hyperosmolar hyperglycemic dehydration can lead to convulsions, coma, and death.

Treatment
Add insulin to the IVH solution.

HYPOGLYCEMIA

Causes
Excessive endogenous insulin production after abrupt termination of IVH solution, or excessive delivery of exogenous insulin

Signs and symptoms
Muscle weakness, anxiety, confusion, restlessness, diaphoresis, vertigo, pallor, tremors, and palpitations

Treatment
If possible, give carbohydrates orally; infuse dextrose 10% in water or administer dextrose 50% in water by I.V. bolus.

FLUID DEFICIT

Causes
Hyperglycemia, vomiting, diarrhea, fistula output, large burns, inadequate fluid replacement, electrolyte imbalance

Signs and symptoms
Fatigue, dry skin and mucous membranes, wrinkled tongue, depressed anterior fontanelle (in infants), tachycardia, tachypnea, decreased urinary output, normal or subnormal temperature, decreased central venous pressure, weight loss, hemoconcentration

Treatment
Increase fluid intake.

Continued

Detecting Complications of Intravenous Hyperalimentation (IVH)

Continued

FLUID EXCESS

Causes
Fluid overload, electrolyte imbalance

Signs and symptoms
Puffy eyelids, peripheral edema, elevated central venous pressure, ascites, weight gain, pulmonary edema, pleural effusion, moist rales

Treatment
Reduce fluid intake.

HYPOKALEMIA

Causes
Muscle catabolism, loss of gastric secretions from vomiting, suction, or diarrhea; may occur when anabolism is achieved with its accompanying intracellular movement of potassium

Signs and symptoms
Malaise, lethargy, loss of deep tendon reflexes, muscle cramping, paresthesia, atrial and ventricular dysrhythmias, decreased intensity of heart sounds, weak pulse, hypotension, and complete heart block

Treatment
Increase potassium intake. A malnourished patient may require an initial dose of 60 to 100 mEq/1,000 calories.

HYPOPHOSPHATEMIA

Causes
Phosphate deficiency; infusion of glucose causes phosphate ions to shift at start of IVH or within 48 hours of inadequate phosphate intake

Signs and symptoms
Serum PO_4 levels less than 1 mg/dl cause lethargy, weakness, paresthesia, and glucose intolerance. Severe hypophosphatemia can cause acute hemolytic anemia, convulsions, coma, and death.

Treatment
Add phosphates to the IVH solution.

Continued

Detecting Complications of Intravenous Hyperalimentation (IVH)
Continued

HYPOCALCEMIA

Causes
Increased doses of phosphates administered to correct hypophosphatemia, without supplemental calcium; hypoalbuminemia or excess free water

Signs and symptoms
Nausea, vomiting, diarrhea, hyperactive reflexes, tingling at fingertips and mouth, carpopedal spasm, dysrhythmias, tetany, and convulsions

Treatment
Add calcium to the IVH solution.

HYPOMAGNESEMIA

Cause
Inadequate intake of magnesium; exacerbated by severe diarrhea and vomiting

Signs and symptoms
Lethargy, tremors, athetoid or choreiform movements, positive Chvostek's or Trousseau's sign, paresthesia, convulsions, and tetany

Treatment
Add magnesium to the IVH solution.

ESSENTIAL FATTY ACID DEFICIENCY

Cause
Absent of inadequate fat intake for an extended period

Signs and symptoms
Alopecia, brittle nails, desquamating dermatitis, increased capillary fragility, indolent wound healing, reduced prostaglandin synthesis, increased platelet aggregation, thrombocytopenia, enhanced susceptibility to infection, fatty liver infiltration, lipid accumulation in pulmonary macrophages, notching of R waves in EKG, growth retardation (in children)

Treatment
For the adult patient, infuse two or three bottles of 10% or 20% fat emulsion daily.

Continued

Detecting Complications of Intravenous Hyperalimentation (IVH)
Continued

ZINC DEFICIENCY

Cause
Altered requirements associated with stress, the degree of intracellular zinc deficit, and induced zinc deficiencies from redistribution during anabolism

Signs and symptoms
Diarrhea, apathy, confusion, depression, eczematoid dermatitis (initially in nasolabial and perioral areas), alopecia, decreased libido, hypogonadism, indolent wound healing, acute growth arrest, and hypogeusesthesia (diminished sense of taste)

Treatment
Add zinc to the IVH solution.

HYPOCUPREMIA

Causes
Long-term IVH without addition of copper sulfate; infection, high-output enterocutaneous fistulas, and diarrhea predispose to copper deficiency

Signs and symptoms
Neutropenia and hypochromic microcytic anemia

Treatment
Add copper to the IVH solution.

Special Consideration

Remember these important points about intravenous hyperalimentation (IVH):
- Know that IVH promotes tissue synthesis, wound healing, and normal metabolic function by providing calories, maintaining positive nitrogen balance, and supplying or replacing needed essential vitamins, electrolytes, and minerals.
- During IVH, watch for possible complications, such as septicemia, fungal infection, air emboli, hemothorax, hydrothorax, pneumothorax, and pleural effusion.
- If you suspect an air embolism, place the patient on his left side in Trendelenburg position.

Understanding Blood Component Therapy

All blood component products are extracted from whole blood, but each has different characteristics. So some blood components treat certain hematologic disorders better than others. The doctor will choose a blood component product based on how well it will treat your patient's condition. For example, if your patient needs volume replenishment quickly, he'll receive a volume expander. If his blood isn't clotting properly, he'll receive a product with clotting factors.

Here's a chart to help you learn more about blood component products and their uses.

WHOLE BLOOD

Contents
• Red blood cells (RBCs), white blood cells (WBCs), platelets, plasma, and plasma clotting factors

Uses
• To restore blood volume and to replenish oxygen-carrying capacity in a patient with massive hemorrhage

Nursing considerations
• Administer through a large-gauge I.V. over 2 to 4 hours, or as ordered.

PACKED CELLS

Contents
• RBCs and 20% plasma
• Less sodium and potassium than whole blood

Uses
• To replenish blood's oxygen-carrying capacity while minimizing risk of fluid overload in patients with severe anemia, slow blood loss, or congestive heart failure

Nursing considerations
• Administer more slowly than whole blood (unless diluted with saline solution).

WASHED CELLS

Contents
• RBCs and 20% plasma
• Fewer WBCs and platelets than packed cells

Uses
• To replenish blood's oxygen-carrying capacity in patients previously sensitized by transfusions

Nursing considerations
• Administer at a slower rate than whole blood (unless diluted with saline solution).

GRANULOCYTES

Contents
• WBCs and 20% plasma

Uses
• To treat life-threatening granulocytopenia (<500/mm³)

Continued

Understanding Blood Component Therapy
Continued

GRANULOCYTES
Continued

Nursing considerations
• Administer rapidly.
• Expect the patient to develop fever, chills, hypertension, or disorientation during transfusion; these are considered to be transfusion reactions.

PLASMA (FRESH-FROZEN)

Contents
• Clotting Factors II, III, V, VII, IX, X, and XIII; fibrinogen; prothrombin; albumin; and globulins
Uses
• To treat patients with clotting factor deficiencies (the only treatment for Factor V deficiency)
• To expand volume
Nursing considerations
• Fresh-frozen plasma takes 20 minutes to thaw, so call the blood bank ahead of time.
• Administer 1 unit over 1 hour.

PLATELETS

Contents
• Platelets, WBCs, and plasma
Uses
• To correct low platelet counts (<10,000/mm³)
Nursing considerations
• Administer 1 unit over 10 minutes.

CRYOPRECIPITATE

Contents
• Factors VIII and XIII and fibrinogen
Uses
• To replace clotting factors in patients with disseminated intravascular coagulation, hemophilia A, von Willebrand's disease, fibronogen deficiency, or Factor XIII deficiency
Nursing considerations
• Administer rapidly *immediately after thawing,* to ensure factor activation.

ALBUMIN (5% AND 25%)

Contents
• 5% and 25% albumin from plasma
Uses
• To replace volume in patients suffering from shock, burns, hypoproteinemia, or hypoalbuminemia
Nursing considerations
• Administer 1 ml/minute or, *if the patient's in shock,* administer rapidly.
• May administer with dextrose 5% in water.

Continued

Understanding Blood Component Therapy
Continued

PLASMA PROTEIN FRACTION

Contents
• 5% albumin and globulin solution in saline solution
Uses
• To expand volume in patients with burns, hemorrhage, or hypoproteinemia
Nursing considerations
• Administer 1 ml/minute.
• Risk of hepatitis or sensitization is low.

PROTHROMBIN

Contents
• Factors II, VII, IX, and X
Uses
• To replace clotting factors in patients with hemophilia B or bleeding secondary to severe liver disease
Nursing considerations
• Prothrombin is used infrequently because of increased hepatitis risk.

Transfusions: Blood Type Compatibility
Precise blood typing and cross matching are essential—if the donor's blood is incompatible with the recipient's, the transfusion can be fatal. In most instances, determining the recipient's blood type and cross matching it with available donor blood take less than 1 hour.

The four blood groups are distinguished by their agglutinogen (antigen in RBCs) and their agglutinin (antibody in serum or plasma).

BLOOD TYPE	AGGLUTINOGEN TYPE	AGGLUTININ TYPE
A	A	Anti-B
B	B	Anti-A
AB	A and B	None
O	None	Anti-A and Anti-B

OTHER CRITICAL CARE CONCERNS

Continued

Transfusions: Blood Type Compatibility *Continued*
The following chart shows the compatible blood groups.

RECIPIENT	A/B	AB	O
DONOR			
A	Yes/No	Yes	No
B	No/Yes	Yes	No
AB	No/No	Yes	No
O	Yes/Yes	Yes	Yes

A New Advance in Blood Replacement
Soon you may see use—particularly in emergencies—of perfluorochemical (Fluosol-DA). Here's how Fluosol compares with blood.

BLOOD	FLUOSOL
• Expands circulating volume	• Expands circulating volume
• Has RBCs and hemoglobin that carry oxygen to ischemic tissues	• Has particles that can infiltrate and carry more oxygen
• Carries 85% of the blood's oxygen no matter how much supplemental oxygen is given	• Can carry extra oxygen when administered with high concentrations of supplemental oxygen
• Provides clotting factors and platelets	• Doesn't provide clotting factors or platelets
• Must be refrigerated, typed, and crossmatched	• Doesn't need to be refrigerated, typed, or crossmatched
• Usually requires no pretreatment	• Requires pretreatment with corticosteroids to prevent reactions
• Is readily available	• Pending FDA approval

Administering Blood Transfusions

As you know, if a blood transfusion's administered improperly, the patient may develop a transfusion reaction. To minimize the risk of reaction and subsequent complications when you transfuse blood, review the procedure outlined here.

Equipment
• Blood administration set with filter and drip chamber
• 250 ml normal saline solution
• Whole blood or selected blood component
• I.V. pole, venipuncture equipment, and 20G—or larger—angiocatheter (if the patient doesn't already have an I.V. line)

Before the procedure
• Explain the procedure to the patient.
• Make sure he's signed a consent form. If the patient's religious beliefs prohibit blood transfusions, make sure you follow your hospital's protocols.
• Take the patient's vital signs to serve as baseline values.
• Check that the blood type ordered is compatible with the patient's blood type.
• Check the doctor's order for specific directions concerning how many units to administer and over how much time.

• Check the patient's history to see if he's had a reaction to a previous transfusion. If so, he has a greater chance of developing a reaction again, so watch him carefully.
• If the patient doesn't have an I.V. line established, see that one is started. Infuse normal saline solution to keep the vein open. Blood is viscous, so avoid using an existing line if the needle or angiocatheter is smaller than 19G.
• Obtain the blood from the blood bank or blood refrigerator *just before administering it.* Remember, red blood cells (RBCs) deteriorate at room temperature.
• Compare chart information—the patient's identification number and blood type—with his compatibility record. Also compare the patient's name and identification number on his wristband with the information on the compatibility record and blood bag. If the patient can speak, ask him to identify himself by his full name.
• Check the expiration date on the blood bag and observe the blood for abnormal color, RBC clumping, gas bubbles, and abnormal cloudiness. If you see any of these return the blood; it may be contaminated or hemolyzed.

Continued

Administering Blood Transfusions
Continued

• Check your hospital's policy for transfusion protocol on how often to take the patient's vital signs during the transfusion and how to dispose of the empty blood bag. Follow this policy to the letter.

• If you're giving whole blood, gently invert the bag several times to mix the cells.

• Prepare for transfusion by letting the blood run through the administration set to expel air from the tubing.

During the procedure
• Keep the patient warm.

• Hang the blood 3' to 4' (about 1 m) above the level of the patient's heart.

• Plug the blood tubing into the port closest to the patient, turn the saline solution off, and begin transfusing the blood slowly, 25 to 30 drops/minute. (He should receive only 50 ml over the first 30 minutes.)

• Remain with the patient and take his vital signs periodically. Watch him for signs of transfusion reaction for the first 15 to 30 minutes. If no signs of reaction appear within that time, adjust the flow clamp to the ordered infusion rate.

• Check the patient after another 15 minutes, then check the patient hourly or according to specific protocol.

After the procedure
• Flush the filter and tubing with normal saline solution if the manufacturer recommends this.

• If you have to give another transfusion, disconnect the set that's hanging and use another set with the next unit.

• If you don't have to give another transfusion, disconnect the blood line and flush the main line with normal saline solution.

• Reconnect the original I.V. or discontinue the saline solution as ordered.

• Record the date and time of the transfusion, the type and amount of blood transfused, the patient's vital signs during the transfusion, and any transfusion reaction and subsequent interventions.

Recognizing Transfusion Reactions

During a blood transfusion, your patient's at risk for developing any of five types of reactions. To learn to recognize them and to intervene appropriately, study this chart.

If your patient develops any sign or symptom of a reaction, immediately follow this procedure:
• Stop the transfusion.
• Change the I.V. tubing to prevent infusing any more blood. Save the tubing and blood bag for analysis.
• Administer saline solution I.V. to keep the vein open.
• Take the patient's vital signs.
• Notify the doctor.
• Obtain urine and blood samples from the patient and send them to the laboratory.
• Prepare for further treatment.

HEMOLYTIC

Signs and symptoms
Chills, fever, low back pain, headache, chest pain, tachycardia, dyspnea, hypotension, nausea and vomiting, restlessness, anxiety, shock

Nursing considerations
• Expect to place the patient in a supine position, with his legs elevated 20° to 30°, and to administer oxygen, fluids, and epinephrine to correct shock.
• Expect to administer mannitol to maintain the patient's renal circulation.
• Expect to insert an indwelling (Foley) catheter to monitor the patient's urinary output (should be about 100 ml/hr).

• Expect to administer antipyretics to lower the patient's fever. If his fever persists, expect to apply a hypothermia blanket or to give tepid sponge or alcohol baths.

PLASMA PROTEIN INCOMPATIBILITY

Signs and symptoms
Chills, fever, flushing, abdominal pain, diarrhea, dyspnea, hypotension

Nursing considerations
• Expect to place the patient in a supine position, with his legs elevated 20° to 30°, and to administer oxygen, fluids, and epinephrine to correct shock.
• Expect to administer corticosteroids.

Continued

Recognizing Transfusion Reactions
Continued

FEBRILE

Signs and symptoms
Range from mild chills, flushing, and fever to extreme signs and symptoms resembling a hemolytic reaction

Nursing considerations
• Expect to administer an antipyretic and an antihistamine for a *mild* reaction.
• Expect to treat a *severe* reaction the same as a hemolytic reaction.

BLOOD CONTAMINATION

Signs and symptoms
Chills, fever, abdominal pain, nausea and vomiting, bloody diarrhea, hypotension

Nursing considerations
• Expect to administer fluids, antibiotics, corticosteroids, vasopressors, and a fresh transfusion.

ALLERGIC

Signs and symptoms
Range from pruritus, urticaria, hives, facial swelling, chills, fever, nausea and vomiting, headache, and wheezing to laryngeal edema, respiratory distress, and shock

Nursing considerations
• Expect to administer parenteral antihistamines or, for a severe reaction, epinephrine or corticosteroids.
• If the patient's only sign of reaction is hives, expect to restart the infusion, as ordered, at a slower rate.

Special Consideration

OTHER
CRITICAL CARE CONCERNS

If the doctor anticipates a transfusion reaction, he may order prophylactic treatment before blood administration. Record the time and date of transfusion reaction, the type and amount of infused blood or blood products, the signs of transfusion reaction in order of occurrence, the patient's vital signs, any specimens that were sent to the laboratory for analysis, any treatment, and patient's response to treatment. If required by your hospital, complete the transfusion reaction form.

—PATRICIA GONCE MILLER, RN, MS

Transfusion Risks: When Administering Massive Amounts

Infusing large amounts of blood naturally carries greater risks than infusing single units. But did you know the complications don't result as much from the large volume as from the necessity for using stored blood? Do what you can to protect your patient against these possible complications. Study this chart, and take the suggested precautions.

BLEEDING TENDENCIES

Cause
Low platelet count in stored blood, causing dilutional thrombocytopenia

Signs and symptoms
Abnormal bleeding, and oozing from raw or cut surfaces

Treatment
Administer platelets, as ordered by doctor.

Prevention
Use only fresh blood (less than 7 days old, if possible).

HYPOCALCEMIA

Cause
A reaction to toxic proportions of citrate, which is used as a preservative in blood. Either the citrate ion combines with calcium, causing a calcium deficiency, or normal citrate metabolism is hindered by hepatic disease.

Signs and symptoms
Tingling sensation in fingers, muscle cramps, convulsions, hypotension, shock, tetany, or cardiac arrest

Treatment
Slowly administer calcium chloride I.V., as ordered by doctor.

Prevention
Monitor calcium levels carefully, especially if patient has hepatic disease. Follow the doctor's orders for treatment. Use only frozen saline-washed cells. As you know, the plasma has been removed from these cells, which lowers the citrate content.

INCREASED OXYGEN AFFINITY

Cause
A decreased level of 2,3,DPG in stored blood, causing an increase in the oxygen's hemoglobin affinity. When that happens, oxygen stays in the patient's bloodstream and isn't released into his tissues.

Signs and symptoms
Depressed respirations, especially in patients with chronic lung disease, who depend on their low oxygen level to breathe.

Treatment
Monitor arterial blood gas measurements, and give respiratory support, as needed.

Prevention
Use only red blood cells or fresh blood, if possible.

Continued

OTHER
CRITICAL CARE CONCERNS

Transfusion Risks: When Administering Massive Amounts
Continued

POTASSIUM INTOXICATION

Cause
An abnormally high potassium level in stored plasma, caused by red blood cell lysis

Signs and symptoms
Renal failure; nausea; diarrhea; vague muscle weakness; slow or irregular heartbeat; paresthesias of hands, face, tongue; EKG changes: tall, peaked T waves

Treatment
Administer hypertonic Kayexalate orally or by enema, as ordered.

Prevention
Use only red blood cells, fresh frozen plasma, or blood stored for less than 7 days, especially if patient has renal failure.

ELEVATED BLOOD AMMONIA LEVEL

Cause
An increased level of ammonia in stored blood

Signs and symptoms
Forgetfulness, confusion

Treatment
Decrease amount of protein in diet. If the doctor orders, give neomycin sulfate (Mycifradin Sulfate*, Neobiotic) when necessary.

*Available in the United States and Canada.

Prevention
Use only red blood cells, fresh frozen plasma, or blood stored less than 7 days, especially if patient has hepatic disease.

HEMOSIDEROSIS

Cause
Increased hemosiderin (iron-containing pigment) from red blood cell destruction

Signs and symptoms
Iron plasma level greater than 200 mg/100 ml

Treatment
Perform a phlebotomy to remove excess iron.

Prevention
Don't administer blood unless it's absolutely necessary.

HYPOTHERMIA

Cause
Large volume of blood administered at too cold a temperature

Signs and symptoms
Decreased temperature, chills, and possible cardiac arrest

Treatment
Call the doctor. Warm the patient with blankets.

Prevention
Warm blood before giving massive transfusion.

Transfusion Risks: Transmittable Diseases

You can never be sure the blood you're infusing is disease-free. This chart will help you identify some of the diseases that can be transmitted by transfusion, tell you how to treat them effectively, and how to help prevent them from occurring in other patients.

HEPATITIS

Cause
Presence of hepatitis B in blood (greatest risk in pooled plasma, fibrinogen, concentrates of Factors VIII and IX; no risk in immune serum, globulin, PPF, normal serum albumin)

Incubation time
2 weeks to 6 months

How to confirm
Make sure the blood is tested for hepatitis B antigens before administering it. Patient will have anorexia, vomiting, abdominal discomfort, enlarged liver, diarrhea, headache, fever, and jaundice.

How to treat
Isolation, gamma globulin therapy, supportive treatment

How to prevent
Select reliable, healthy blood donors. Conduct epidemologic follow-ups of suspected cases to potential carriers. Conduct radioimmunoassays for hepatitis B on all donor blood products. Make sure blood is tested for the Australia antigen.

SYPHILIS

Cause
Spirochetemia caused by *Treponema pallidum*

Incubation time
4 to 18 weeks

How to confirm
Check blood for syphilis with a serologic test, but don't consider results absolutely reliable.

How to treat
Administer penicillin therapy.

How to prevent
Don't administer blood unless it's been tested and refrigerated for at least 2 days at 39.2° F. (4° C.).

VIRAL SYNDROME

Cause
Presence of cytomegalovirus (CMV) or Epstein-Barr virus in blood

Incubation time
2 to 5 weeks

How to confirm
The patient will show signs of fever, hepatitis, atypical lymphocytosis, and rash.

How to treat
No specific therapy.

How to prevent
Select only those donors who are free from recent viral symptoms.

Understanding Autotransfusion

You're assessing a boy's chest wound when you detect signs and symptoms of shock: blood loss, decreased blood pressure, and increased heart rate. The doctor examines the boy, tells you he has a hemothorax, and gives an order to prepare him for autotransfusion.

Using this procedure, the doctor will remove the blood that's filled the boy's pleural space. Then he'll reinfuse it into the boy's system—quickly—to treat the shock. Why not do a regular transfusion? Because the boy's shock condition allows no time to type and cross match his blood.

Here's how autotransfusion works and what you need to know to assist with it.

How it works

As you may know, autotransfusion collects, filtrates, and reinfuses the patient's own blood. It helps treat massive blood loss (1,000 ml or more) from hemothorax as well as heart or great vessel injuries. To use autotransfusion, the chest cavity can't be contaminated with gastrointestinal contents such as those from wounds of the esophagus, stomach, or bowel. The wound can't be more than 4 hours old, and the blood can't have been hemolyzed.

The procedure works as follows:

• The vacuum system sucks shed blood through the sterile chest tube and into the sterile canister liner.
• The canister contains citrate-phosphate-dextrose to prevent clotting of collected blood, and a fine-screen filter to remove microaggregated platelets, air bubbles, fat, and debris.
• The liner's removed from the canister when reinfusion is necessary or when 1,900 ml of blood have been collected.
• A microemboli filter's attached to the I.V. line. Blood is quickly reinfused through transfusion tubing, using gravity drip. Infusion pumps can be used for rapid infusion.

Nursing interventions

• Before you assist with autotransfusion, be sure you're familiar with the procedure and the equipment.
• Maintain sterility of the equipment and the system during the procedure.
• Make sure all the connections on the equipment are secure.
• Change the microemboli filter after collecting 1,900 ml of blood.
• Carefully document all therapeutic measures, times, blood volumes lost and replaced, and serial assessments of the patient's condition.

Using the Sengstaken-Blakemore Tube to Control Esophageal Bleeding

To help control bleeding when your patient has ruptured esophageal varices, the doctor may ask you to help him insert a Sengstaken-Blakemore (S-B) tube. Why? Because inflation of the tube's balloons will compress the varices and temporarily restrict bleeding.

The S-B tube has an esophageal balloon and a gastric balloon. Each of the three lumens attached to the tube has a specific function: One inflates the esophageal balloon, one inflates the gastric balloon, and one suctions gastric contents below the gastric balloon.

Preparation

The doctor may ask you to prepare the S-B tube for insertion by chilling and lubricating it. He may also ask you to check for air leaks in the balloons by inflating them and holding them under water: if no bubbles appear, the balloons are intact.

Before the tube's inserted, elevate the head of the pa-tient's bed to a semi-Fowler position (unless he's in shock). And, as always, explain the procedure to him and provide emotional support.

Insertion and inflation

As the doctor inserts the S-B tube, encourage the patient to breathe through his mouth and to sip some water. Initial confirmation of tube placement involves injecting air into the gastric port, while auscultating the patient's abdomen, and aspirating gastric contents. Do this if the doctor orders it. The doctor will immediately order an X-ray to confirm the tube's position, but he won't wait for it. Instead, he'll proceed to inflate the gastric balloon with 250 to 500 cc of air.

When the gastric balloon's inflated, double-clamp its air intake port, and tape the nasal cuff in place on the S-B tube. This will minimize pressure on the patient's nostril. (To keep the patient comfortable with the tube in place,

Continued

Using the Sengstaken-Blakemore Tube to Control Esophageal Bleeding
Continued

consider having him wear a football helmet—if one's available and the doctor okays its use. Then you can tape the tube to the helmet's face guard.)

Next, lavage the patient's stomach with normal or iced saline solution, as ordered, and attach the gastric suction port to an intermittent suction apparatus (Gomco). This prevents nausea and allows blood evacuation from the stomach and continuous observation of gastric contents.

Now, the doctor will inflate the esophageal balloon. When he's finished, double-clamp the esophageal air intake port. To prevent accumulation and aspiration of esophageal secretions above the esophageal balloon, the doctor may ask you to insert a nasogastric tube through the patient's other nostril into his esophagus. Or he may insert it himself. (If you're using a Minnesota tube, be aware that it has a fourth lumen for this purpose.) Attach the port

to suction, as ordered.

Nursing considerations
- Check and record the patient's vital signs frequently. Be especially alert for signs and symptoms of esophageal rupture, shock, and increased bleeding and respiratory difficulty.
- *Keep a pair of scissors taped to the head of the patient's bed.* Then you'll be ready, if the patient develops acute respiratory distress, to grasp the tube at the nostril, to cut across it to deflate both balloons, and to remove it without delay.
- Maintain balloon pressures at the required levels—check the pressure every 4 to 6 hours. As ordered, deflate the balloons periodically, to prevent necrosis of the stomach and esophagus. Be alert to recurrence of bleeding or aspiration of stomach contents—have suction equipment available and be ready to reinflate the balloon if needed.
- Maintain suction, as ordered, on the tube's gastric and esophageal aspiration ports.

Continued

OTHER
CRITICAL CARE CONCERNS

Using the Sengstaken-Blakemore Tube to Control Esophageal Bleeding
Continued

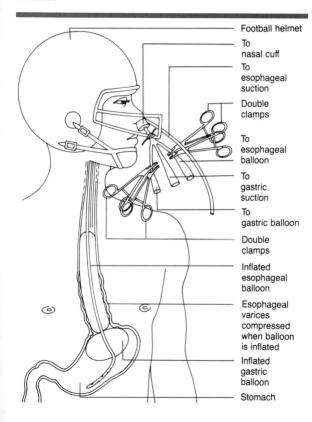

Football helmet

To nasal cuff

To esophageal suction

Double clamps

To esophageal balloon

To gastric suction

To gastric balloon

Double clamps

Inflated esophageal balloon

Esophageal varices compressed when balloon is inflated

Inflated gastric balloon

Stomach

Normal Tube Drainage

TUBE	SUBSTANCE	AMOUNT DAILY
Foley	Urine	500 to 2,500 ml
Gastrostomy	Gastric contents	Up to 1,500 ml
Hemovac	Wound drainage	Depends on operative procedure
Ileal conduit	Urine	500 to 2,500 ml
Ileostomy	Small bowel contents	Minimal to 500 ml
Miller-Abbott	Intestinal	Up to 3,000 ml
Nasogastric	Gastric contents	Up to 1,500 ml
T-Tube	Bile	500 ml
Suprapubic	Urine	500 to 2,500 ml
Ureteral	Urine	750 ml (30 ml/hr)

COLOR	ODOR	CONSISTENCY
Yellow	Ammonia	Watery
Pale yellow-green	Sour	Watery
Varies with procedure	None	Variable
Yellow	Ammonia	Watery, with some mucus initially
Brown	Sour, fecal	Initially serous, mucuslike, liquid stool
Dark green to brown	Fecal	Thick
Pale yellow-green	Sour	Watery
Bright yellow to dark green	Acrid	Thick
Yellow	Ammonia	Watery
Yellow	Ammonia	Watery

Using Traction to Immobilize a Spinal Cord–Injured Patient

Your spinal cord–injured patient will have to be immobilized for as long as 1 to 3 months. For this, his doctor may use skull tongs, such as Gardner-Wells or Vinke, or halo-vest traction. Here's what you should know about these two types of skeletal traction units—and about caring for an immobilized patient.

SKULL TONGS

Used to immobilize the patient's cervical spine after fracture or dislocation, invasion by tumor or infection, or surgery

Nursing considerations
• Reassure the patient and explain the procedure to him.
• Assess his neurologic signs, as ordered, with particular emphasis on motor function. Notify the doctor *immediately* if the patient experiences decreased sensation or increased loss of motor function: this may indicate *spinal cord trauma.*

• Be alert for signs and symptoms of loosening pins: redness, swelling, and complaints of persistent pain and tenderness. (Causes of loosening pins include infection, excessive traction force, and osteoporosis.)
• If the pins pull out, immobilize the patient's head and neck and call the doctor.
• Take action to prevent pressure sores. Remember, inadequate peripheral circulation can cause sores within 6 hours.
• Make sure the traction weights are hanging freely to maintain proper traction force. *Never add or subtract weights unless the doctor orders it.* (Inappropriate weight adjustment may cause neurologic impairment.)

Continued

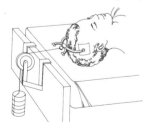

Using Traction to Immobilize a Spinal Cord–Injured Patient
Continued

HALO-VEST TRACTION

Used to immobilize the patient's head and neck after cervical spine injury (allows greater mobility than skull tongs; carries less risk of infection)

Nursing considerations
• Reassure the patient and explain the procedure to him.
• Assess his neurologic signs, as ordered, with particular emphasis on motor function.

Notify the doctor *immediately* if the patient experiences decreased sensation or increased loss of motor function: this may indicate *spinal cord trauma*.
• Check the pin sites and use cleansing procedures, as ordered.
• Obtain an order for an analgesic if your patient complains of headache after the doctor retightens the pins.
• Never lift the patient using the device's bars.

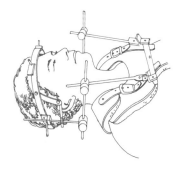

Types of Traction

Mechanical traction exerts a pulling force on a part of the body—usually the spine, the pelvis, or the long bones of the arms and legs. It can be used to reduce fractures, to treat dislocations, to correct or prevent deformities, to improve or correct contractures, or to decrease muscle spasms. Depending on the injury or condition, an orthopedist may order skin or skeletal traction. Applied directly to the skin and thus indirectly to the bone, skin traction is ordered when a light, temporary, or non-continuous pull is required. Contraindications for skin traction include a severe injury with open wounds, an allergy to tape or other skin traction equipment, circulatory disturbances, dermatitis, and varicose veins. In skeletal traction, an orthopedist inserts a pin or wire through the bone and attaches the traction equipment to the pin or wire to exert a direct, constant, longitudinal pull. Indications for skeletal traction include fractures of the tibia, femur, and humerus. Such infections as osteomyelitis contraindicate skeletal traction.

Nursing responsibilities for this procedure include setting up a basic or Balkan traction frame. The design of the patient's bed usually dictates whether to use a claw clamp or I.V.-post-type frame. (However, the claw-type Balkan frame is rarely used.) Setup of the specific traction can be done by a specially trained nurse or by the doctor. Instructions for setting up these specific traction units usually accompany the equipment. After the patient is placed in the specific type of traction as ordered by the orthopedist, the nurse is responsible for preventing complications from immobility; for routinely inspecting the equipment; for adding traction weights, as ordered; and, in patients under skeletal traction, for monitoring the pin insertion sites for signs of infection.

TYPE	DESCRIPTION AND COMMON USES
Buck's extension 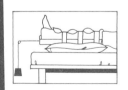	• *Skin traction* usually applied to leg by weight attached to spreader bar below foot, and pulling force is applied with the leg in a straight line. • Pillow placed under leg keeps pressure off heel. • *Uses:* dislocated hip after reduction; hip fractures before surgery; after total hip replacement; locked knee; fractured femur before surgical reduction; irritated hip or knee joint.

Continued

Types of Traction
Continued

TYPE	DESCRIPTION AND COMMON USES

Dunlop's

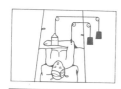

- Applies lateral traction to elbow; temporary, used for children.
- Using *skin traction,* shoulder is abducted 90° and elbow extended in 45° position *to stretch biceps muscle.*
- Uses two pulling forces: one applied laterally to forearm by skin traction, the other downward by sling hanging from distal portion of upper arm. Forces act on elbow from two directions with different magnitudes, causing pull in a third direction.
- *Uses:* transcondylar and supracondylar fractures of humerus; contracture of elbow.

Overhead (90°-90°)

If applied to arm, upper arm is perpendicular to body, elbow is flexed 90°, and forearm is supported by sling suspended from overhead pulley.
- Usually used with *skeletal application,* with pin insertion through olecranon.
- *Uses:* fracture of humerus or elbow; fracture or injury of shoulder; may also be applied to legs for displaced fractured femur in children, or for lower back pain.

Russell's

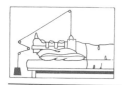

- *Skin traction* to affected leg and sling placed under knee.
- Uses two pulling forces: one applied by double-pulley system at foot, and the other applied upward by sling under knee attached to single overhead pulley.
- *Uses:* congenital hip dislocation; hip fracture; after total hip replacement; fractured femur; disease of hip or knee.

Continued

Types of Traction
Continued

TYPE	DESCRIPTION AND COMMON USES

Sidearm

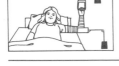

- May be applied by skin or skeletal traction.
- For lateral-longitudinal traction of humerus, shoulder is abducted 90° and externally rotated, elbow is flexed 90° and kept perpendicular to bed.
- *For skin traction,* separate wraps are used on upper arm and forearm.
- *Skeletal traction* applied by pin through olecranon, with forearm traction by adhesive straps and elastic bandage.
- *Uses:* fractures, dislocations, and other pathologies of upper arm and shoulder; tissue injury around elbow (skin traction).

Balanced suspension with Thomas splint

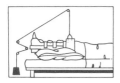

- May be used with skin and skeletal traction to suspend leg in splint and permit patient to move freely in bed.
- Distribution of weights exerts traction force, provides countertraction, and suspends leg.
- Pearson attachment is sometimes used with Thomas splint to support lower leg off bed, allowing knee flexion.
- *Uses:* fractures of femoral shaft, hip, and/or lower leg.

Traction Frame

Claw-type basic frame:
Claw attachments secure
the uprights to the foot-
board and headboard.

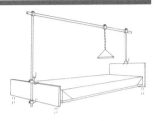

I.V.-type basic frame: I.V.
posts, placed in I.V. hold-
ers, support the horizontal
bars across the foot and
head of the bed. These
horizontal bars then sup-
port the two uprights.

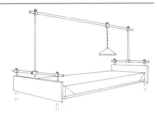

I.V. Balkan frame: I.V.
posts and horizontal bars,
secured in the same man-
ner as those for the I.V.
basic frame, support four
uprights.

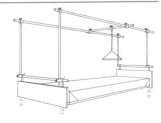

Turning Your Patient on a Stryker Frame

Frames and beds
To care for a patient with spinal cord injuries who's immobilized on a frame or bed, you'll need to know the following: how to maintain proper spinal alignment; how to prevent further spinal cord damage; and how to promote healing of his bony injury. Additionally, you must take measures to prevent skin breakdown and contracture deformities.

Stryker frame
A patient with severe neck or back injuries may be immobilized on a Stryker frame. Make sure you explain the purpose of the frame to your patient and his family; it will probably seem frightening to them. Unless your patient's prepared, he may fear falling when he's turned.

The Stryker frame uses an anterior and a posterior frame with canvas covers and thin padding over each. The frames, which are supported on a movable cart, have a pivot

apparatus at each end. This allows you to change the patient's position to either prone or supine without altering his alignment.

To do this properly, follow the manufacturer's instructions or your hospital's procedure manual.

Further tips: Before turning your patient, secure any equipment he may have, such as I.V.s, Foley catheter, or respirator tubing to make sure it'll easily turn with him.

Some patients prefer to be turned more quickly than others. Place your patient's preference on his care plan along with the turning schedule.

• To prevent malalignment, check the equipment periodically and tighten the lacing of the canvases.

• To protect your patient's skin, place a foam mattress or padding on both frames and cover it with sheepskin.

• To aid in maintaining proper alignment, use a footboard, hand roll, bolsters, and splints as required.

Continued

Turning Your Patient on a Stryker Frame
Continued

1

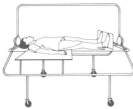

Proper patient alignment;
supine position

2

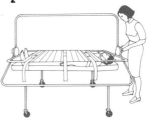

Frame secured with safety
straps over patient

3

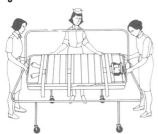

Turning the patient

4

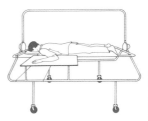

Turn accomplished.
Proper patient alignment;
prone position

Setup for Continuous Slow Ultrafiltration

In continuous slow ultrafiltration, blood enters the ultrafiltration system from the arterial end of the patient's shunt and passes through a red (arterial) port where it is heparinized by way of continuous heparin infusion. Blood then flows through the artificial kidney for ultrafiltration

removal, passes through the blue (venous) port, and reenters the patient through the venous arm of the shunt. The ultrafiltration line attaches to a urinary drainage bag. A screw clamp on the line may be used to regulate the ultrafiltrate flow.

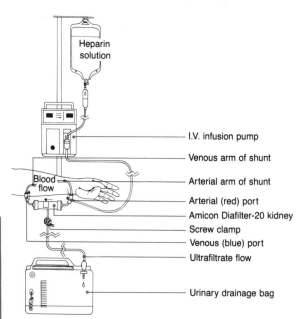

Heparin solution

I.V. infusion pump

Venous arm of shunt

Arterial arm of shunt

Blood flow

Arterial (red) port

Amicon Diafilter-20 kidney

Screw clamp

Venous (blue) port

Ultrafiltrate flow

Urinary drainage bag

Guide to Hemodialysis Complications

INTERNAL HEMORRHAGE

Possible cause
• Excessive heparinization
Nursing considerations
• Decrease initial heparin dose, or use minimal or regional heparinization.
• Observe patient for signs of internal bleeding: apprehension; restlessness; pale, cold, clammy skin; excessive thirst; decreased blood pressure; rapid, weak, and thready pulse; increased respirations; decreased temperature.
• Doctor may order blood transfusions.

EXTERNAL HEMORRHAGE

Possible cause
• Line disconnection
Nursing considerations
• Observe for leakage.
• Keep clamps ready in case any line disconnects.
• Keep blood pressure cuff nearby to use as a tourniquet.

AGGRAVATED ANEMIA

Possible cause
• Blood loss in hemodialyzer

lines and equipment
Nursing considerations
• Doctor may order blood transfusions, folic acid, and iron.

HEPATITIS

Possible cause
• Blood transfusion with infected blood
Nursing considerations
• Take care not to infect patient when performing blood transfusions and dialysis: wear gloves, particularly if you have an open wound; cap all needles; observe strict aseptic technique.
• If patient has hepatitis, keep him in isolation during hemodialysis.
• Patient should be tested every 4 weeks for hepatitis; staff should be tested every 3 months.

DIALYSIS DISEQUILIBRIUM SYNDROME

(headache, fatigue, muscle agitation, twitching, and confusion, possibly leading to grand mal seizure)

Continued

Guide to Hemodialysis Complications
Continued

DIALYSIS DISEQUILIBRIUM SYNDROME
Continued

Possible cause
● Rapid shift of fluid and electrolyte levels
Nursing considerations
● Slow blood flow rate during hemodialysis.
● Inform doctor immediately; he may order diazepam (Valium*), or phenytoin sodium (Dilantin*), or discontinue therapy.
● Doctor may order other treatment, for symptoms.

HYPOTENSION

Possible causes
● Septic shock
● Reduced blood volume from extracorporeal circulation
● Poor cardiac output
Nursing considerations
● Place the patient supine.
● Infuse normal saline solution, as necessary, to restore blood volume.
● Doctor may order mannitol, plasma, or albumin infusion.
● Check blood pressure every 10 minutes until stable.

CARDIAC DYSRHYTHMIA OR ANGINA

Possible causes
● Rapid shift of fluid and electrolyte levels
● Reduced blood volume from extracorporeal circulation
● Reduced hematocrit level
Nursing considerations
● If hyperkalemia is the cause, doctor will order sodium polystyrene sulfonate.
● If decreased blood volume is the cause, the doctor will order blood transfusions.
● Doctor may order antiarrhythmics, for example, lidocaine or procainamide hydrochloride.

MUSCLE CRAMPING

Possible cause
● Rapid shift of fluid and electrolyte levels
Nursing considerations
● Doctor may order normal saline solution infused with 100 ml 25% mannitol, 10 ml 23% sodium chloride, or 50 ml dextrose 50%.

Continued

Guide to Hemodialysis Complications
Continued

LOWER BACK PAIN

Possible cause
• Blood flow rate too rapid at start of hemodialysis
Nursing considerations
• Reduce initial blood flow rate.
• Doctor may order diphenhydramine hydrochloride (Benadryl*).

AIR EMBOLISM

Possible causes
• Insufficient blood flow
• I.V. bag empty
• Loose connections
Nursing considerations
• Monitor blood flow rate carefully.

• Hang bags rather than bottles of dialysate, because bags are less likely to admit air into tubing.
• Clamp I.V. line before bag empties.
• Make sure tubing connections are secure.
• If patient's blood pressure falls rapidly, if he has a weak, rapid pulse, and if he is cyanotic, turn him on his left side and lower the head of the bed. This position will help keep on the right side of his heart any air that's entered, so the pulmonary artery can absorb air bubbles. Notify the doctor immediately.
*Available in the United States and Canada.

Special Consideration

Make sure you complete each step in the dialysis procedure accurately. *Overlooking a single step or performing it incorrectly can cause unnecessary blood loss or inefficient treatment due to poor clearances or inadequate fluid removal.* Ultimately, failure to perform accurate hemodialysis therapy can lead to patient injury and even death. Throughout hemodialysis, carefully monitor vital signs. Take blood pressure readings at least hourly and, if needed, as often as every 15 minutes. Monitor the patient's weight regularly *to ensure adequate ultrafiltration during treatment.* Perform periodic tests for clotting time on both the patient's blood samples and dialyzer samples.

OTHER
CRITICAL CARE CONCERNS

INDEX

INDEX

INDEX

INDEX